2nd edition

BOC
STUDY GUIDE

HISTOTECHNOLOGY

Certification Examinations
Histotechnician (HT)
Histotechnologist (HTL)

Oversight Editors

Freida L Carson, PhD, MASCP, HT(ASCP)
Department of Pathology (retired)
Baylor University Medical Center
Dallas, Texas

Glenda F Hood, MEd, HT(ASCP)
Histotechnology Program Director (retired)
Tarleton State University
Fort Worth, Texas

Publishing Team

Erik N Tanck & Annabelle Ulalulae (production)
Joshua Weikersheimer (publishing direction)

Notice

Trade names for equipment and supplies described are included as suggestions only. In no way does their inclusion constitute an endorsement of preference by the Author or the ASCP. The Author and ASCP urge all readers to read and follow all manufacturers' instructions and package insert warnings concerning the proper and safe use of products. The American Society for Clinical Pathology, having exercised appropriate and reasonable effort to research material current as of publication date, does not assume any liability for any loss or damage caused by errors and omissions in this publication. Readers must assume responsibility for complete and thorough research of any hazardous conditions they encounter, as this publication is not intended to be all inclusive, and recommendations and regulations change over time.

PRESS

Printed in the United States of America

24 23 22 21 20

ISBN 978-089189-6494   ©ASCP 2016

Table of Contents

To the examinee,

Certification is an important first step in your professional career. It is my hope that you find your career in laboratory medicine a rewarding one.

Good luck on your certification exam and on your future endeavors.

– Patricia A Tanabe, MPA, MLS(ASCP)^{CM}
Executive Director, Board of Certification

Acknowledgment

Our thanks to Diane L Sterchi, MS, HT/HTL(ASCP), who reviewed and edited questions for this book.

Preface

The *Board of Certification Study Guide for Histotechnology Certification Examinations 2e* contains over 1,100 multiple choice questions. Unique to this study guide is the differentiation of questions appropriate for both the entry level histotechnicians and histotechnologists and the levels from questions that are appropriate for the entry level histotechnologists **only** (marked with an asterisk). The questions in this edition are arranged in chapters which correspond to the major content areas on the examination. Within each chapter, the questions are further grouped by topic. New to this edition are short answer explanations and references for each practice question. Questions with images will appear as they would on the certification examination. Laboratory results will be presented in both conventional and SI units.

The practice questions are presented in a format and style similar to the questions included on the Board of Certification certification examinations. **Please note:** *None* **of these questions will appear on any Board of Certification examination.**

This book is not a product of the Board of Certification; rather, it is a product of the ASCP Press, the independent publishing arm of the American Society for Clinical Pathology. Use of this book does not ensure passing of an examination. The Board of Certification's evaluation and credentialing processes are entirely independent of this study guide; however, this book should significantly help you prepare for your BOC examination.

ISBN 978-089189-6494   ©ASCP 2016

The Importance of Certification, CMP, Licensure & Qualification

The practice of modern medicine would be impossible without the tests performed in the laboratory. A highly skilled medical team of pathologists, specialists, laboratory scientists, technologists, technicians, and phlebotomists works together to determine the presence or absence of disease and provides valuable data needed to determine the course of treatment.

Today's laboratory uses many complex, precision instruments and a variety of automated and electronic equipment. However, the success of the laboratory begins with the laboratorians' dedication to their profession and willingness to help others. Laboratorians must produce accurate and reliable test results, have an interest in science, and be able to recognize their responsibility for affecting human lives.

Role of the ASCP Board of Certification

Founded in 1928 by the American Society of Clinical Pathologists (ASCP—now, the American Society for Clinical Pathology), the Board of Certification is considered the preeminent certification agency in the US and abroad within the field of laboratory medicine. Composed of representatives of professional organizations and the public, the Board's mission is to: *"Provide excellence in certification of laboratory professionals on behalf of patients worldwide."*

The Board of Certification consists of more than 100 volunteer technologists, technicians, phlebotomists, laboratory scientists, physicians, and professional researchers. These volunteers contribute their time and expertise to the Board of Governors and the Examination Committees. They allow the BOC to achieve the goal of excellence in credentialing medical laboratory personnel in the US and abroad.

The Board of Governors is the policymaking governing body for the Board of Certification and is composed of 23 members. These 23 members include technologists, technicians, and pathologists nominated by the ASCP and representatives from the general public as well as from the following societies: the American Association for Clinical Chemistry, the AABB, American Society for Microbiology, American Society for Clinical Laboratory Science, the American Society of Cytopathology, the American Society of Hematology, the American Association of Pathologists' Assistants, Association of Genetic Technologists, the National Society for Histotechnology, and the Clinical Laboratory Management Association.

The Examination Committees are responsible for the planning, development, and review of the examination databases; determining the accuracy and relevancy of the test items; confirming the standards for each examination and performing job or practice analyses.

Certification

http://www.ascp.org/certification

Certification is the process by which a nongovernmental agency or association grants recognition of competency to an individual who has met certain predetermined qualifications, as specified by that agency or association. Certification affirms that an individual has demonstrated that he or she possesses the knowledge and skills to perform essential tasks in the medical laboratory. The ASCP Board of Certification certifies those individuals who meet academic and clinical prerequisites and who achieve acceptable performance levels on examinations.

In 2004, the ASCP Board of Certification implemented the **Credential Maintenance Program** (CMP), which mandates participation every 3 years for newly certified individuals in the US. The goal of this program is to demonstrate to the public that laboratory professionals are performing the appropriate and relevant activities to keep current in their practice. Please follow the steps outlined on the website to apply for CMP and retain your certification (http://www.ascp.org/CMP).

United States Certification
http://www.ascp.org/certification

To apply for a Certification Examination follow these step-by-step instructions:

1 Identify the examination you are applying for and determine your eligibility.

2 Gather your required education and experience documentation.

3 Apply for the examination online and pay by credit card, PayPal, check, or money order.

4 Submit required documentation.

5 Upon notification of your eligibility, schedule your examination at a Pearson Professional Center. Visit the Pearson site (http://www.pearsonvue.com/ascp) to identify a location and time that is convenient for you to take your ASCP examination.

International Certification
http://www.ascp.org/certification/International

ASCP offers its gold standard credentials in the form of international certification (ASCP[i]) to eligible individuals. The ASCP[i] credential certifies professional competency among new and practicing laboratory personnel in an effort to contribute globally to the highest standards of patient safety. Graduates of medical laboratory science programs outside the United States are challenged with content that mirrors the standards of excellence established by the US ASCP exams. The ASCP[i] credential carries the weight of over 80 years of expertise in clinical laboratory professional certification. Please visit the website to view the following:

1 Website information translated into a specific language.

2 Current listing of international certifications.

3 Eligibility guidelines.

4 Step-by-step instructions to apply for international certification.

State Licensure
http://www.ascp.org/licensure

State Licensure is the process by which a state grants a license to an individual to practice their profession in the specified state. The individual must meet the state's licensing requirements, which may include examination and/or experience. It is important to identify the state and examination to determine your eligibility and view the steps for licensure and/or certification. For a list of states that require licensure, please go to the website (http://www.ascp.org/statelicensureagencies).

The ASCP Board of Certification (BOC) examinations have been approved for licensure purposes by the states of California and New York. The BOC examinations also meet the requirements for all other states that require licensure.

Qualification
http://www.ascp.org/qualification

A qualification from the Board of Certification recognizes the competence of individuals in specific technical areas. Qualifications are available in laboratory informatics, immunohistochemistry, laboratory safety, cytometry, and apheresis. To receive this credential, candidates must meet the eligibility requirements and successfully complete an examination (QIHC, QLS, QCYM, QIA) or a work sample project (QLI). Candidates who complete the Qualification process will receive a Certificate of Qualification, which is valid for 3 years. The Qualification may be revalidated every 3 years upon receipt of completed application and fee. (Documentation of acceptable continuing education may be requested.)

ISBN 978-089189-6494   ©ASCP 2016

Preparing for & Taking the BOC Certification Examination

Begin early to prepare for the Certification Examination. Because of the broad range of knowledge and skills tested by the examination, even applicants with college education and those completing formal laboratory education training programs will find that review is necessary, although the exact amount will vary from applicant to applicant. Generally, last minute cramming is the least effective method for preparing for the examination. The earlier you begin, the more time you will have to prepare; and the more you prepare, the better your chance of successfully passing the examination and scoring well.

Study for the Test

Plan a course of study that allows more time for your weaker areas. Although it is important to study your areas of weakness, be sure to allow enough time to review all areas. It is better to spend a short time studying every day than to spend several hours every week or 2. Setting aside a regular time and a special place to study will help ensure studying becomes a part of your daily routine.

Study Resources

http://www.ascp.org/studymaterials

Content Guidelines

http://www.ascp.org/contentguidelines

The Board of Certification has developed content guidelines to delineate the content and tasks included in its tests. Current Content Guidelines for the Histotechnologist (HTL) and Histotechnician (HT) examinations as well as other certification examinations offered by the ASCP BOC are available online.

Study Guide

The questions in this study guide are in a format and style similar to the questions on the Board of Certification examinations. The questions are in a multiple choice format with 1 best answer. Work through each chapter and answer all the questions as presented. Next, review your answers against the answer key. Review the answer explanation for those questions that you answered incorrectly. Lastly, each question is referenced if you require further explanation.

Textbooks

The references cited in this study guide (see p 307) identify many useful textbooks. The most current reading lists for most of the examinations are available on the ASCP's website (http://www.ascp.org/readinglists). Textbooks tend to cover a broad range of knowledge in a given field. An added benefit is that textbooks frequently have questions at the end of the chapters that you can use to test yourself should you need further clarification on specific subject matter.

Online practice tests

http://www.ascp-practice.com

The online practice test is a subscription product. It includes 90-day online access to the practice tests, comprehensive diagnostic scores, and discussion boards. If you are an institutional purchaser that would like to pay by check or purchase order (minimum of 20 tests to use a check or purchase order), please download the order form from the website. Content-specific online practice tests can be purchased online.

Taking the Certification Examination

The ASCP Board of Certification uses the format of computer adaptive testing (CAT) for all certification examinations. With CAT, when a person answers a question correctly, the next test question has a higher level of difficulty. The difficulty level of the questions presented to the examinee continues to increase until a question is answered incorrectly. Then an easier question is presented. In this way, the test is tailored to the individual's ability level

Each question in the test bank is calibrated for level of difficulty and is classified by content area. The content area aligns with the examination specific content outline. The examinee must answer enough questions correctly to achieve a measure above the pass point in order to successfully pass the certification examination. There is no set number of questions one must answer to pass, nor is there a set percentage one must achieve to pass. If at the end of the exam the examinee's score is above the pass point, then he or she passes the exam.

All examinations (with the exception of phlebotomy (PBT) and donor phlebotomy (DPT)) are scheduled for 2 hours and 30 minutes and have 100 questions. The PBT examinations is scheduled for 2 hours and has 80 questions, and the DPT examination is scheduled for 2 hours and 30 minutes and has 90 questions. Your preliminary test results (pass/fail) will appear on the computer screen immediately upon completion of your examination. Notification to view your examination scores will be emailed within 4 business days after your examination, provided that the BOC has received all required application documents. Examination results cannot be released by telephone under any circumstances.

Your official examination score report will indicate a "pass" or "fail" status and the scaled score on the total examination. A scaled score is mathematically derived (in part) from the raw score (number of correctly answered questions) and the difficulty level of the questions. Because each examinee has taken an individualized examination, scaled scores are used so that all examinations may be compared on the same scale. The minimum passing score is 400. The highest attainable score is 999.

If you were unsuccessful in passing the examination, your scaled scores on each of the subtests will be indicated on the report as well. These subtest scores cannot be calculated to obtain your total score. These scores are provided as a means of demonstrating your areas of strengths and weaknesses in comparison to the minimum pass score.

Fixation

The following items have been identified as appropriate for both entry level histotechnicians and histotechnologists.

1   An example of an additive fixative is one that contains:

   a picric acid
   b acetic acid
   c ethyl alcohol
   d acetone

2   When compared with tissue fixed in formalin, tissue fixed in zinc-formalin will show:

   a better ultrastructural preservation
   b decreased immunoreactivity
   c increased enzyme activity
   d superior nuclear detail

3   Microscopic examination of an H&E stained section fixed in formalin shows marked nuclear bubbling. One most often sees this artifact if the specimen is processed following:

   a incomplete fixation
   b prolonged fixation
   c microwave fixation
   d frozen sectioning

4   Microscopic evaluation of H&E stained sections from a surgically removed small bowel specimen shows an absence of much of the epithelium in otherwise normal tissue. This most likely resulted from:

   a mechanical trauma
   b delayed fixation
   c ulceration
   d poor choice of fixative

5   A specimen of kidney must be shipped to another city for immunofluorescence studies. The specimen should be placed in:

   a saline
   b Michel solution
   c buffered formalin
   d Orth solution

6   A certain project requires a fixative that contains acetic acid yet stabilizes erythrocyte membranes. One fixative that could be used is:

   a Zenker solution
   b Bouin solution
   c Gendre solution
   d Hollande solution

7   When the microwave oven is used for fixation, the most critical factor is the:

   a preparation of the formalin solution
   b use of glass containers
   c control of the temperature
   d osmolality of the fixation solution

8   To adequately remove the calcium from a specimen containing areas of microcalcification, the tissue could be fixed in:

   a Hollande solution
   b neutral buffered formalin
   c B-5 solution
   d Zamboni solution

9   Which of the following fixatives contains copper acetate?

   a Hollande
   b Bouin
   c Gendre
   d Zamboni

10   A specimen is submitted with the statement that it was fixed in formalin. Microscopic sections show marked lysis of erythrocytes. This indicates that the fixative most likely was:

   a prepared with too much formalin
   b buffered above neutrality
   c acidified with acetic acid
   d not formalin

11   Fixatives are classified as additive because of the:

   a addition of several chemicals to the solution
   b addition, or binding of the fixative to tissue proteins
   c additional reactions occurring with longer fixation
   d additional reactive tissue sites available for dye binding

12   Kidney biopsy tissue has been fixed in phosphate-buffered glutaraldehyde for 2 hours and then placed in phosphate buffer solution. If a portion of this tissue is processed for light microscopy, sections would most likely show:

   a very poor glomerular preservation
   b decreased uptake of hematoxylin
   c lysis of cytoplasmic elements
   d nonspecific PAS staining

13   Uric acid crystals are preserved ONLY when tissue is fixed in:

   a absolute alcohol
   b neutral buffered formalin
   c Orth solution
   d Zamboni solution

14   Improper preservation of tissue will result if there is:

   a a delay in fixation
   b rapid penetration of the fixing fluid
   c prolonged storage following formalin fixation
   d rapid dehydration, clearing, embedding, and sectioning

15   A good fixative will:

   a render cell constituents soluble
   b minimize differences in tissue refractive indices
   c protect tissue against alteration during subsequent processing
   d minimally affect tissue metabolic processes

16   The function of methanol in commercial formalin solutions is to:

   a retard the polymerization of formaldehyde
   b prevent the formation of formic acid
   c stabilize the formalin at a basic pH
   d permit room temperature storage of formalin

17   The problem shown in this image is the result of:

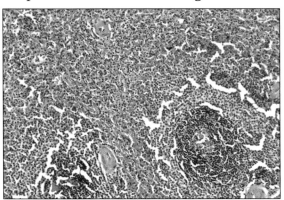

   a incomplete fixation
   b excessive dehydration
   c incomplete clearing
   d poor paraffin infiltration

18   In electron microscopy, Zamboni fluid, glutaraldehyde, and osmium tetroxide function as:

   a dehydrating agents
   b clearing agents
   c embedding media
   d fixative solutions

19   Tissue will remain unfixed if placed in:

   a potassium dichromate
   b sodium borate
   c osmium tetroxide
   d zinc chloride

20   Bouin solution is contraindicated for:

   a small tissue biopsies
   b tissue intended for subsequent trichrome stains
   c tissue to be stained by the Feulgen reaction
   d routine tissue sections

21   Formalin pigment can be removed from tissue sections by treatment with 10%:

   a hydrochloric acid in 70% alcohol
   b nitric acid in 70% alcohol
   c sulfuric acid in 70% alcohol
   d ammonium hydroxide in 70% alcohol

ISBN 978-089189-6494   ©ASCP 2016

22   Stock neutralized formalin is prepared in the laboratory by storing the solution over a layer of calcium carbonate. The solution withdrawn from this stock container will:

     a become acidic
     b become alkaline
     c remain neutral
     d exhibit metachromasia

23   Microscopic evaluation reveals a poorly stained H&E section of spleen. These results will be difficult to remedy if the problem is:

     a poor fixation
     b improper sectioning
     c poor staining
     d incorrect section placement

24   To make a 10% formalin solution, how many mL of water should be added to 300 mL of 37% to 40% formaldehyde solution?

     a 1,800
     b 2,500
     c 2,700
     d 3,600

25   One action of acetic acid is to:

     a exert a shrinking effect on tissue
     b render nucleoprotein acidophilic
     c form salt linkages between protein chains
     d coagulate nucleoproteins

26   Aldehyde fixatives are used for electron microscopy preparations because they:

     a are readily available
     b visibly stain tissue
     c preserve cell ultrastructure
     d coagulate tissue lipids

27   A fixative containing potassium dichromate:

     a is suitable when histochemical techniques are planned
     b will result in excellent subsequent silver staining
     c is preferred for the preservation of argentaffin cells
     d will make tissue more receptive to eosin staining

28   If mercuric chloride is used alone for fixation, it will:

     a leave tissue proteins uncoagulated
     b produce a very acidic solution
     c penetrate poorly and cause excessive shrinkage
     d decrease tissue affinity for stains

29   Tissue stored for long periods of time in unbuffered formalin or in acetate formalin may show brown, crystalline pigment in stained sections. To remove this pigment prior to staining it is necessary to treat the microscopic section with:

   a saturated alcoholic picric acid
   b alcoholic lithium chloride
   c iodine and sodium thiosulfate
   d potassium permanganate and oxalic acid

30   For good fixation of tissue with osmium tetroxide for electron microscopy, it is recommended that the tissue segment be no larger than:

   a 1 mm^3
   b 2 mm^3
   c 1 cm^3
   d 2 cm^3

31   The tissue shown in this image is:

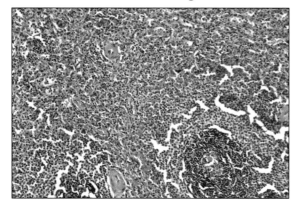

   a liver
   b kidney
   c spleen
   d lymph node

32   Following fixation with Bouin solution, tissue should be washed with:

   a absolute alcohol
   b 50% to 70% alcohol
   c 20% to 40% alcohol
   d saline solution

33   The PTAH staining technique would require postfixation, or mordanting, if the tissue were originally fixed in:

   a Bouin
   b Zenker
   c Gendre
   d formalin

  ISBN 978-089189-6494   ©ASCP 2016

34   The problem seen in this image is known as:

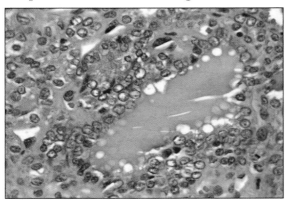

    a cell shrinkage
    b smudgy nuclei
    c pyknotic nuclei
    d nuclear bubbling

35   Absolute ethanol is a poor choice for the fixation of:

    a glycogen
    b pigments
    c lipids
    d blood smears

36   Which of the following fixatives may give false positive results in some carbohydrate techniques?

    a neutral buffered formalin
    b Bouin solution
    c Gendre solution
    d glutaraldehyde

37   It is necessary to adjust the pH of most formalin solutions because of the presence of:

    a methanol
    b formic acid
    c paraformaldehyde
    d carbon dioxide

38   The rate of fixation varies with the fixative and also with the:

    a time placed in the fixative of choice
    b expected completion time of the report
    c anticipated special stains needed
    d temperature of the fixative solution

39   Carnoy solution is recommended for the preservation of:

    a acid-fast bacilli
    b nucleic acids
    c lipids
    d red blood cells

40   Which of the following factors affects fixation for light microscopy the least?

    a temperature
    b volume ratio
    c penetration rate
    d pH

41   Formalin pigment is generally created in tissues fixed in formalin when the pH:

    a rises above 6
    b falls below 6
    c is buffered to neutrality
    d is 7.2

42   Very bloody cytology smears are often treated with:

    a 10% formalin
    b Hollande solution
    c Clark solution
    d acetone

43   Glyoxal is one of the newer fixatives which has the added advantage of:

    a ability to crosslink
    b rapidity of action
    c enhanced staining
    d preservation of erythrocytes

44   If a tissue section was fixed in a solution different from that required for a
    staining procedure, microscopic sections frequently can be stained anyway if they
    are:

    a soaked in a solution of lithium carbonate prior to staining
    b revitalized by washing in a solution of sodium bisulfite
    c postfixed in the appropriate fixative prior to staining
    d treated with hydrogen peroxide

45 The nuclear problem seen in this image is:

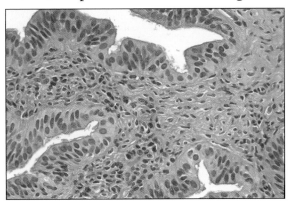

    a understained chromatin
    b cell shrinkage
    c smudgy nuclei
    d nuclear bubbling

46 Fixation in Bouin solution is:

    a recommended for the Feulgen reaction
    b excellent for ultrastructural preservation
    c the cause of considerable swelling of tissue
    d frequently used for endocrine tissues

47 B-5 fixative contains:

    a mercuric chloride, sodium acetate, and glacial acetic acid
    b mercuric chloride, potassium dichromate, and glacial acetic acid
    c mercuric chloride, sodium acetate, and 37% to 40% formaldehyde
    d mercuric chloride, potassium dichromate, and 37% to 40% formaldehyde

48 Pigment caused by mercury-containing fixatives can be removed from tissues by:

    a saturated alcoholic picric acid
    b iodine-sodium thiosulfate
    c washing in running water
    d potassium hydroxide in water

49 Which of the following fixatives has a mordanting effect on tissue?

    a Carnoy solution
    b 10% calcium formalin
    c absolute alcohol
    d Bouin solution

50   Tissue should be placed in a fixative solution immediately after removal from the body to:

   a prevent decomposition due to enzymatic activity
   b permit the dehydrant to function properly
   c inhibit crosslinking of tissue proteins
   d stabilize tissue carbohydrates

51   Calcium-formalin fixative is recommended for the BEST preservation and subsequent demonstration of:

   a glycogen
   b phospholipids
   c amyloid
   d estrogen receptors

52   For most fixatives, the volume of fixing fluid in relation to the volume of tissue should be:

   a 2 to 5 times
   b 6 to 9 times
   c 10 to 14 times
   d 15 to 20 times

53   Ultrastructural preservation will be very poor following fixation in:

   a Zamboni PAF
   b 2% buffered glutaraldehyde
   c osmium tetroxide
   d 10% aqueous formalin

54   Glyoxal is a/an:

   a aliphatic hydrocarbon
   b aromatic hydrocarbon
   c dialdehyde
   d ketone

55   Zinc-formalin fixatives:

   a give poor ultrastructural preservation
   b can be used to preserve enzymes
   c result in poor nuclear detail
   d will not coagulate tissue proteins

56   Zamboni PAF refers to a fixative containing:

   a potassium dichromate, acetic acid, and formaldehyde
   b potassium aluminum sulfate and paraformaldehyde
   c buffered picric acid and formaldehyde
   d picric acid, acetic acid, and formaldehyde

57 The problem seen in this image most likely could have been prevented by:

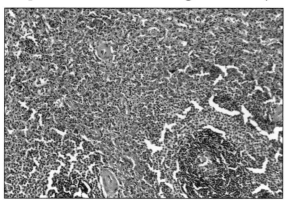

   a immediate and prolonged fixation
   b less processing time
   c increased paraffin infiltration
   d better microtomy technique

58 The preferred fixative when tissue is to be stained for the presence of simple fats is:

   a Zenker
   b Helly
   c Hollande
   d neutral buffered formalin

59 Fixation of cytology smears should occur within:

   a 1-2 seconds
   b 10-15 seconds
   c 40-45 seconds
   d 1 minute

60 When osmium tetroxide is used as a fixative in histology, it:

   a destroys lipids
   b interferes with staining
   c leaves tissue very soft
   d distorts cell membranes

61 The breakdown of tissue due to enzyme activity is called:

   a polymerization
   b putrefaction
   c autolysis
   d osmosis

62 The fixative of choice for the demonstration of a gouty tophus is:

  a neutral buffered formalin
  b absolute alcohol
  c Bouin solution
  d Zenker solution

63 A good fixative for routine use is one that:

  a makes tissue more permeable to fluids
  b is hypotonic to the tissue constituents
  c enhances putrefaction of tissue components
  d promotes tissue autolysis

64 A pigment caused by chromate-containing fixatives can be prevented by treating the tissue prior to processing with:

  a running water
  b iodine
  c picric acid
  d potassium permanganate

65 When fixing tissue for electron microscopy with formaldehyde or glutaraldehyde, the preservation of ultrastructure depends upon all of the following EXCEPT the:

  a pH
  b time and temperature
  c concentration and purity of the reagent
  d type of tissue

66 Formic acid present in commercial formalin solutions may:

  a facilitate pigment formation
  b precipitate hemosiderin
  c promote staining
  d cause tissue shrinkage

67 Carnoy solution is a combination of which of the following chemicals?

  a absolute alcohol, acetone, and glacial acetic acid
  b cedarwood oil, absolute alcohol, and glacial acetic acid
  c acetone, chloroform, and absolute alcohol
  d chloroform, glacial acetic acid, and absolute alcohol

68 When using a nonimmunologic stain for chromaffin granules, it is necessary to fix the tissue in a:

  a mercury fixative
  b primary chromate fixative
  c formalin fixative
  d picric acid fixative

69   When liver tissue is fixed with 2% to 3% glutaraldehyde:

   a glycogen is dissolved
   b the penetration rate is very rapid
   c a chemical reaction occurs with lipids
   d the ultrastructure is preserved

70   A poor fixative is characterized by:

   a the absence of shrinking or swelling of tissue
   b inactivation of tissue enzymes
   c slow tissue penetration
   d the absence of distortion or dissolution

71   The problem seen in this image possibly could have been prevented by:

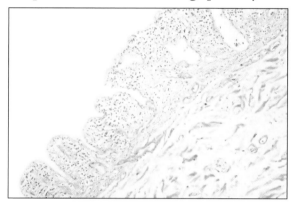

   a buffering the formaldehyde solution
   b immediate contact with fixative solution
   c grossing the specimen more carefully
   d better processing protocol

72   Bouin solution contains all of the following EXCEPT:

   a picric acid
   b absolute alcohol
   c 37% to 40% formaldehyde
   d glacial acetic acid

73   Coagulant fixatives:

   a change the spongework of proteins into a mesh-like network
   b produce fewer artifacts than noncoagulant fixatives
   c act very slowly to fix tissues
   d leave protein linkages unaffected

74   The breakdown of tissue by bacterial action is called:

   a autolysis
   b putrefaction
   c denaturation
   d oxidation

75   When ultrastructural preservation is of the utmost importance, the fixative used should have a pH of:

   a 6.8 to 7.0
   b 7.2 to 7.4
   c 7.6 to 7.8
   d 8.0 to 8.2

76   A fixative component that produces a diffuse brownish black pigment is:

   a picric acid
   b osmium tetroxide
   c mercuric chloride
   d acetic acid

77   For the BEST preservation of staining properties during long-term storage, tissues should be stored in:

   a buffered formalin
   b 10% formal-saline
   c 70% ethanol
   d Zamboni solution

78   Ethanol is useful as a fixative because it:

   a crosslinks proteins
   b increases tissue basophilia
   c prevents tissue shrinkage
   d preserves glycogen very well

79   The nuclear problem seen in this image is most often attributed to:

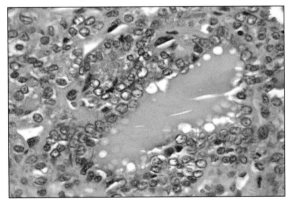

   a delay in fixation
   b incomplete fixation
   c overdehydration
   d poor paraffin infiltration

80   To prevent the formation of formalin pigment in tissues, formalin should be:

     a heated
     b cooled
     c buffered
     d acidified

81   Which of the following fixatives should be used for specimens that may NOT be processed for several days?

     a 10% neutral buffered formalin
     b Bouin solution
     c Helly solution
     d Zenker solution

82   A biopsy that was placed in water by mistake is submitted to the laboratory. This mistake most likely will cause:

     a mushy sections
     b swollen and ruptured cells
     c hardening of the tissue
     d no appreciable changes

83   Sections of a breast carcinoma were fixed in a saline solution in the microwave oven. Microscopic examination of H&E stained sections show marked pyknotic, overstained nuclei. The staining results were most likely caused by the:

     a use of saline for fixation
     b solution temperature exceeding 68°C
     c use of plastic containers in the microwave
     d presence of carcinoma in the breast tissue

84   An unknown pigment in a tissue section that can be bleached with a saturated alcoholic solution of picric acid is most likely:

     a melanin pigment
     b formalin pigment
     c hemosiderin
     d mercury pigment

85   The formaldehyde in Helly solution:

     a causes reduction of some chemicals in the solution
     b coagulates and denatures tissue proteins
     c prevents turbidity and precipitate formation
     d eliminates the need for postfixation washing

86   Formaldehyde solutions for routine use are most commonly buffered by:

   a monobasic and dibasic phosphates
   b sodium acetate and acetic acid
   c s-collidine and hydrochloric acid
   d sodium barbitol and sodium hydroxide

87   The preferred fixative for the image seen below is:

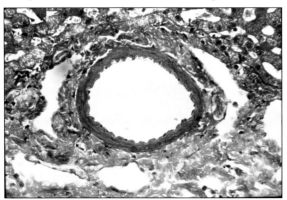

   a 10% neutral buffered formalin
   b alcohol
   c Clark solution
   d Bouin solution

88   One characteristic of Zamboni fixative is that it:

   a does not stabilize cellular proteins
   b may be used for electron microscopy
   c is easily destroyed by tissue fluids
   d must be followed by osmium tetroxide

89   The BEST fixative for blood smears is:

   a Bouin solution
   b Carnoy solution
   c B-5 solution
   d methanol

90   When used as a secondary fixative, osmium tetroxide should be:

   a used after lead citrate
   b heated prior to use
   c combined with alcohol
   d used under a chemical hood

91   Which of the following fixatives is recommended for use in lipid histochemistry?

   a Zenker solution
   b acetone
   c formalin-saline
   d calcium-formalin

92   In the Cajal method for demonstrating astrocytes, sections of brain should be
     fixed in formalin that contains:

     a sodium acetate
     b ammonium bromide
     c mercuric chloride
     d calcium chloride

93   Hollande solution is a modification of which of the following fixatives?

     a Helly solution
     b Orth solution
     c Carnoy solution
     d Bouin solution

94   Tissue fixed in which of the following solutions must be posttreated for mercuric
     chloride pigment?

     a B-5
     b Zamboni
     c Carnoy
     d Orth

95   Acetone is recommended for the primary fixation of:

     a prostate tissue for immunohistochemistry
     b kidney tissue for fluorescent antibody techniques
     c muscle tissue for enzyme histochemistry
     d brain tissue for the diagnosis of rabies

96   Fresh, unfixed tissue can be stored safely for a short time by:

     a keeping it in a freezer
     b wrapping it in saline-moistened gauze and refrigerating it
     c placing it in physiologic saline at room temperature
     d leaving it in a dry specimen container on the counter with a note to the
          histologist

97   The nuclei in this image indicate:

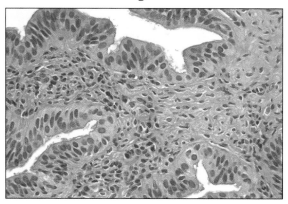

    a excellent chromatin demonstration
    b the use of old hematoxylin
    c incomplete fixation
    d overhydration

98   One characteristic of Bouin solution is that it:

    a penetrates poorly
    b destroys delicate structures
    c mordants connective tissue stains
    d preserves erythrocytes

99   The fixation of tissue by physical methods can be accomplished by the use of:

    a microincineration
    b microwaves
    c frozen sections
    d alcohol

100   Fixation in Carnoy solution will result in:

    a swelling of the tissue
    b preservation of most cytoplasmic structures
    c superior staining of amyloid with Congo red
    d good preservation of red blood cells

101   The recommended fixative for tissue suspected of containing spirochetes is:

    a 10% neutral buffered formalin
    b Bouin solution
    c Zenker solution
    d Helly solution

102 Which of the following is frequently added to formalin solutions to help preserve immunoreactivity?

   a glycerin
   b sodium acetate
   c zinc salts
   d chromates

103 Which of the following fixatives is contraindicated when silver stains are to be done for *Helicobacter pylori*?

   a glutaraldehyde
   b neutral buffered formalin
   c glyoxal
   d Bouin solution

104 A fixative used for the preservation of some enzymes is:

   a Bouin solution
   b B-5 solution
   c acetone
   d isopropanol

105 A common reason for adding acetic acid to fixatives is to:

   a coagulate proteins
   b reduce shrinkage
   c preserve carbohydrates
   d change the pH

106 Formaldehyde acts as a fixative by:

   a uncovering acid groups
   b coagulating proteins
   c crosslinking proteins
   d rupturing peptide linkages

107 If it is known prior to fixation that a distinction must be made between collagen and muscle, the preferred fixative is:

   a neutral buffered formalin
   b Orth fluid
   c absolute alcohol
   d Bouin fluid

108 Bouin fixation is contraindicated for Feulgen stains because during fixation:

   a nucleoproteins are precipitated
   b nuclei are excessively hydrolyzed
   c nucleoproteins are crosslinked
   d RNA is dissolved

109 When using Bouin fixative, the shrinking effect produced by one component is balanced by the swelling effect of:

   a formalin
   b acetic acid
   c osmium tetroxide
   d potassium dichromate

110 10% formalin is equivalent to what percent paraformaldehyde solution?

   a 40
   b 10
   c 4
   d 1

111 To obtain the same nuclear detail characteristic of cytologic preparations, which of the following percentage concentrations of isopropyl alcohol may be substituted for 95% ethyl alcohol?

   a 70
   b 80
   c 90
   d 100

112 Which of the following renders fat insoluble for subsequent processing?

   a picric acid
   b osmium tetroxide
   c chloroform
   d formaldehyde

113 The presence of acetic acid in fixatives produces:

   a cell shrinkage
   b red cell destruction
   c protein coagulation
   d lipid preservation

114 Microscopic review of a formalin fixed tissue section demonstrates a fine, brown-black artifactual pigment. This artifact most likely could have been prevented by:

   a placing the tissue in formalin immediately after removal
   b preparing the solution just before use
   c washing the tissue after fixation
   d making the solution neutral

115 When osmium tetroxide is used as a fixative for paraffin embedding, it:

   a must be used after a primary fixative
   b should be used on very thin sections
   c should be made hypotonic to tissue
   d must be made basic

116 Which of the following fixative components produces shrinkage and penetrates poorly:

    a glacial acetic acid
    b mercuric chloride
    c potassium dichromate
    d ethanol

117 The component in Bouin solution that causes tissue shrinkage is:

    a picric acid
    b acetic acid
    c mercuric chloride
    d potassium dichromate

118 Which of the following fixatives should be selected when it is desirable to preserve erythrocytes in tissue?

    a Clark
    b Bouin
    c Carnoy
    d B-5

119 A tissue section reveals a dark brown microcrystalline pigment which is birefringent. To remove this pigment, the section should be treated with an alcoholic solution saturated with:

    a sodium thiosulfate
    b oxalic acid
    c picric acid
    d hydrochloric acid

120 Shrinkage and distortion of tissue is greatest following fixation in:

    a Bouin solution
    b Zamboni solution
    c absolute alcohol
    d 10% neutral buffered formalin

121 Tissue to be stained by the Warthin-Starry technique should be fixed in:

    a Zenker fluid
    b saturated mercuric chloride
    c formalin
    d osmium tetroxide

122   Because of the location of the pigment, it is most likely:

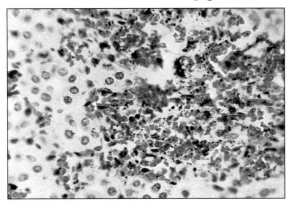

   a formalin
   b mercury
   c chromate
   d melanin

123   The tissue shown in the image below:

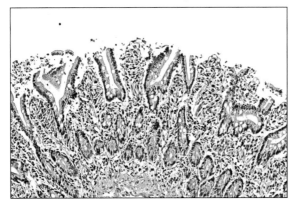

   a esophagus
   b stomach
   c small intestine
   d colon

124   When fat needs to be preserved, the fixative of choice is:

   a formalin
   b Zenker solution
   c Carnoy solution
   d Bouin solution

125   Picric acid was used alone as a fixative for a section of liver. The tissue most likely will show:

   a extreme swelling
   b excessive hardening
   c decreased uptake of eosin
   d hydrolyzed nucleic acids

126 The primary purpose of fixation is the:

   a preservation of carbohydrates
   b coagulation of lipids
   c removal of tissue fluids
   d stabilization of proteins

127 Clark solution lyses erythrocytes because it contains:

   a formalin
   b picric acid
   c acetic acid
   d chloroform

128 The tissue component most affected by the problem shown in the image below is called the:

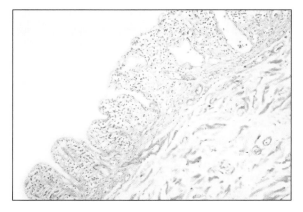

   a lamina propria
   b muscularis
   c epithelium
   d adventitia

The following items (*) have been identified as more appropriate for entry level histotechnologists.

*129 Microscopic examination of a PAS stained section reveals marked nonspecific staining. This could be caused by fixation in:

   a Bouin solution
   b Gendre solution
   c 10% neutral buffered formalin
   d glutaraldehyde solution

*130 The pathologist is sure that urate crystals were present in a tissue biopsy and should therefore be present in the H&E stained section, but polarization of the tissue is negative. This could possibly result from the:

 a application of the wrong stain for demonstration
 b poor clearing and infiltration of the biopsy
 c fact that urate crystals are not birefringent
 d use of a water-based fixative

*131 Formaldehyde reacts primarily with which of the following protein groups?

 a COOH
 b C=O
 c NH_2
 d N=N

*132 During embedding, a white deposit is noted on several of tissues. The tissues had been fixed in zinc-formalin, transferred to phosphate-buffered formalin, dehydrated with 65%, 95%, and absolute alcohols, and cleared with xylene. One possible explanation of the white deposit could be that the tissue was:

 a left in the zinc-formalin too long
 b fixed in incompatible fixatives
 c improperly washed between different formalin fixatives
 d not dehydrated appropriately for the method of fixation

*133 Electron micrographs of a tissue section reveal electron-lucent membranes. This most likely indicates that:

 a fixation was done in Bouin solution
 b the osmolality of the fixative was incorrect
 c the specimen was not postfixed in osmium tetroxide
 d sections were stained with uranyl acetate

*134 Michel medium is:

 a used for transporting unfixed tissue
 b indicated for long-term storage of fixed tissue
 c a fixative with limited use
 d an antigen retrieval solution

*135 Microscopic evaluation of H&E stained sections from a surgically removed, formalin fixed small bowel specimen shows an absence of much of the epithelium in otherwise normal tissue. This could most likely be prevented in the future by:

 a opening the specimen and adding fixative upon receipt
 b avoiding the use of forceps during the dissection
 c allowing the specimen to fix for 48 hours
 d increasing the percentage of formalin in the solution

*136 Recently a laboratory's primary fixative has been changed from neutral buffered formalin to an alcohol-based fixative promoted for antigen preservation. A marked difference in H&E staining is noted, with a marked increase in eosin uptake. These most likely results from the new fixative:

    a creating a different tissue isoelectric point
    b blocking protein precipitation
    c generating more negative charges
    d increasing crosslinking of the amino group

*137 Microscopic evaluation of an H&E stained section of small intestine fixed in 10% neutral buffered formalin shows a complete absence of the surface epithelium and poor cellular detail in the lamina propria. This is most likely the result of:

    a autolysis
    b mechanical trauma
    c antemortem changes
    d prolonged fixation

*138 The problem seen on the section below is most frequently seen in which of the following specimens:

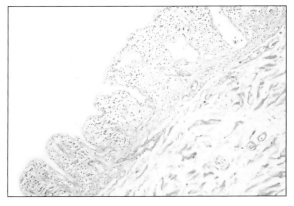

    a colonoscopy
    b post-mortem
    c surgical removal
    d endoscopic biopsy

*139 When sucrose is used to treat tissue for enzyme histochemical studies:

    a cell membranes are mobilized
    b frozen sectioning is very difficult
    c the tissue must be removed after a brief period of treatment
    d the solution should contain 30% sucrose and 1% gum acacia

*140 Kidney tissue has been submitted in Michel medium for immunofluorescence studies. Before the histotechnologist performs the required studies, the tissue should be:

    a washed in PBS containing 10% sucrose
    b frozen immediately upon receipt
    c placed in an aldehyde fixative
    d refrigerated

*141 An isotonic solution for human tissue has an osmolality of approximately:

    a 500 milliosmols
    b 340 milliosmols
    c 260 milliosmols
    d 150 milliosmols

*142 Marked distortion of architecture and predominantly pyknotic nuclei are noted on H&E stained sections of kidney tissue. The tissue was fixed in the microwave in a saline solution. This problem could most likely have been prevented by:

    a changing the processing schedule
    b using another fixative solution
    c carefully controlling the temperature
    d using longer fixation times

*143 Paraffin blocks containing tissue fixed in Bouin solution are retrieved from storage after several years. New sections are cut and stained with H&E, and no nuclear staining is present, although the nuclei of the original slides were well stained. To prevent this from happening in the future on tissue to be stored, one must:

    a neutralize the picric acid before processing
    b be sure that the pH of the Bouin solution is at neutrality
    c make certain that the formalin does not contain formic acid
    d store the blocks in a facility with a maximum temperature of 20°C

*144 Microscopic examination of an H&E stained section fixed in formalin shows nuclear bubbling. This could most likely be avoided in the future by:

    a extending the time of fixation
    b fixing at refrigerator temperatures
    c changing the pH of the fixative
    d decreasing the osmolality of the fixative

*145 During the examination of an electron microscopy print of normal kidney, it is noted that the usual cellular morphology appears disrupted. A possible cause of the problem is that primary fixation occurred in osmium tetroxide for:

    a 1 minute
    b 30 minutes
    c 1 hour
    d 12 hours

*146 Which of the following fixatives is stable at room temperature?

    a Karnovsky paraformaldehyde-glutaraldehyde
    b 2% to 3% glutaraldehyde
    c Zamboni PAF
    d 1% buffered osmium tetroxide

*147 The paraformaldehyde in Zamboni PAF solution must be heated to 60°C prior to adding the 1 M NaOH in order to:

    a dissociate the paraformaldehyde
    b purify the glutaraldehyde
    c polymerize the glutaraldehyde
    d eliminate the gasses present

*148 Prior to processing, tissue fixed in glutaraldehyde for electron microscopy should be:

    a postfixed in formaldehyde
    b rinsed with gum sucrose solution
    c postfixed in osmium tetroxide solution
    d rinsed with an alcohol buffer solution

*149 Poor fixation of electron microscopy specimens is often indicated by the appearance of:

    a evenly dispersed ground substance
    b stabilized cytoplasmic proteins
    c disrupted mitochondrial membranes
    d unaltered nuclear and cytoplasmic membranes

*150 Formalin pigment may be removed from microscopic sections by treating them with:

    a Lugol iodine and sodium thiosulfate
    b potassium permanganate
    c dilute acetic acid
    d potassium hydroxide in 70% alcohol

*151 Fixatives that tend to mask antigenic sites and hamper immunohistochemical localization of antigens contain:

    a mercury
    b phosphates
    c aldehydes
    d alcohol

*152 Microscopic examination of an H&E stained section of fallopian tube reveals very muddy appearing nuclei with no visible chromatin pattern. This is most likely the result of fixation that was?

   a incomplete
   b delayed
   c prolonged
   d appropriate

*153 In immuno-electron microscopy (IEM), a fixative other than osmium tetroxide is used because osmium would:

   a blacken the tissue
   b block entrance of the gold label
   c destroy the antigenicity of the sample
   d decrease membrane preservation

*154 The difference between Orth and Helly solutions is that ONLY Helly contains:

   a formaldehyde
   b potassium dichromate
   c mercuric chloride
   d acetic acid

*155 A small biopsy is submitted with a request for "stat" acid-fast and fungus stains. The tissue should be fixed in:

   a Zenker solution
   b Carnoy fluid
   c B-5 fluid
   d buffered formalin

*156 A microwave oven can be used for fixation because it:

   a causes crosslinking of proteins
   b induces physical fixation
   c increases tissue basophilia
   d inactivates enzymes with beta radiation

*157 Unstained slides from B-5-fixed tissue should be treated with which of the following before staining?

   a lithium carbonate
   b potassium iodide
   c sodium bisulfite
   d iodine

ISBN 978-089189-6494   ©ASCP 2016

*158 Microscopic evaluation of a tissue section reveals a brown pigment lying on top of the tissue. Adjacent sections are treated with: 1. iodine and sodium thiosulfate 2. potassium ferrocyanide and hydrochloric acid 3. saturated alcoholic solution of picric acid. All sections still show the brown pigment. This pigment could have resulted from improper washing following fixation in:

   a Zenker fluid
   b formalin
   c B-5 fluid
   d Bouin fluid

*159 A possible rhabdomyosarcoma has been fixed in 10% neutral buffered formalin. For the nonimmunohistochemical stains needed to confirm this tumor, microscopic sections should be:

   a prepared as frozen sections
   b treated with acetone before staining
   c mordanted in another fixative before staining
   d deparaffinized with xylene-peanut oil mixture

*160 Close examination of the image below reveals a problem that most likely could have been prevented by:

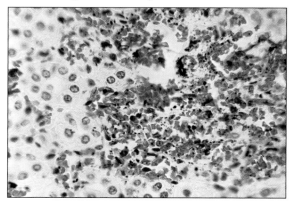

   a washing with running water after fixation
   b neutralizing the tissue before processing
   c ensuring the use of buffered formalin
   d processed on a short cycle

*161 When osmium tetroxide is used on a kidney biopsy for ultrastructural studies, the time of fixation:

   a is not critical
   b should be one hour or less
   c is prolonged because of tissue density
   d depends on the fixative concentration

*162 Helly fixative prepared 3 weeks previously is now discolored and turbid. The most likely reason for this is:

 a the presence of acetic acid in the fixative
 b improper solution buffering
 c the premature addition of formaldehyde
 d chemical oxidation

*163 A stained microscopic section shows marked lysis of erythrocytes and the presence of a brown crystalline pigment. These results indicate that of the following, the fixative was most likely:

 a glutaraldehyde
 b glyoxal
 c acetic acid-formalin
 d methacarn

*164 A small amount of white precipitate is noticed in the bottom of the laboratory's stock 37% to 40% formaldehyde container. The most appropriate action is to:

 a discard the solution
 b disregard the precipitate
 c acidify the solution slightly
 d add methanol to the solution

*165 Acetone can be used to fix tissue for the demonstration of:

 a myelin sheaths
 b phospholipids
 c oxidoreductases
 d cell surface antigens

*166 A tissue block of unfixed hemorrhagic spleen is fixed for 24 hours in formalin that was prepared 6 months previously. Subsequent H&E stained sections show a granular black pigment on the surface of the tissue. This problem can most likely be prevented in the future by:

 a washing the tissue prior to fixation
 b ensuring that the formalin contains buffering reagents
 c using an iodine solution on the processor
 d using only freshly prepared solutions

*167 If the tissue is fixed in formalin, postfixation is critical for a nonimmunohistochemical special stain used in the diagnosis of which of the following tumors?

 a liposarcoma
 b fibrosarcoma
 c neurosarcoma
 d rhabdomyosarcoma

*168 The problem shown below most likely could have been prevented by:

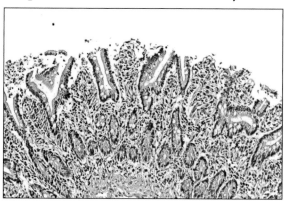

  a more careful grossing technique
  b using a different fixative solution
  c immediate contact with the fixative solution
  d decreasing the flotation bath temperature

*169 A gouty tophus is seen in a fresh tissue specimen. The ideal fixative for the crystals which may be occurring with this condition is:

  a buffered formalin
  b Bouin fluid
  c absolute alcohol
  d Orth fluid

*170 To ensure adequate fixation, a colon polyp measuring approximately 2 × 2 × 3 cm should be placed in, at the minimum, what volume of fixative?

  a 2.4 mL
  b 24 mL
  c 240 mL
  d 2400 mL

*171 A characteristic of acetone fixation is that:

  a glycogen is removed from tissues
  b enzymes are removed from tissues
  c the tissues are overhardened
  d antigen-antibody reactions are destroyed

*172 A wet tissue sample has been requested for electron microscopy. All available tissue has been fixed in Bouin solution, washed, and stored in 70% alcohol. Electron microscopy on the tissue would show:

  a good fixation of nucleoproteins
  b well preserved organelles
  c some shrinkage of the nucleolus
  d inadequately preserved ultrastructures

*173 A surgical specimen is obtained from a patient with a diagnosis of probable metastatic malignant melanoma. The choice of fixatives should be compatible with the use of which of the following special stains or diagnostic procedures?

    a colloidal iron
    b immunohistochemistry
    c immunofluorescence
    d digestion procedures

*174 A section of tendon sheath has been fixed in 10% neutral buffered formalin for 24 hours, routinely processed, and embedded in paraffin. The demonstration of urate crystals on sections from this block:

    a should be performed after postfixation
    b will be best with a fluorescence technique
    c must be performed on air-dried sections
    d will not be possible due to improper fixation

*175 Clark solution differs from Carnoy solution in that only Carnoy contains:

    a absolute alcohol
    b acetic acid
    c chloroform
    d glyoxal

*176 A section of healthy adrenal gland to be used as a control for chromaffin granules is fixed in osmium tetroxide for 8 hours. When examined microscopically, no granules are demonstrated. This problem can be resolved in the future by:

    a washing the tissue before staining
    b selecting another tissue for the control
    c using another fixative
    d increasing the fixation time

*177 An aqueous fixative MUST be chosen for sections that require:

    a the preservation of lipids
    b rapid sample fixation
    c maximum hardening
    d preservation of amyloid

*178 For HER2 testing, it is recommended that fixation be no less than:

    a 2 hours
    b 6 hours
    c 12 hours
    d 48 hours

*179 Tissues that undergo the most rapid autolysis are rich in:

   a connective tissue
   b enzymes
   c blood supply
   d bacteria

*180 Pap smears that have been fixed with a spray fixative are submitted to the laboratory. The smears are stained without another treatment. The most likely result will be

   a excellent cytologic detail
   b the loss of cells from the slide
   c cells showing air-drying artifact
   d nuclei that appear foggy and lack detail

*181 The problem shown below most likely can be prevented in the future by:

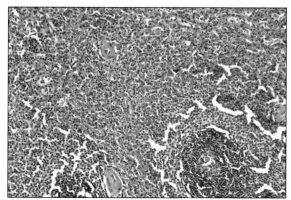

   a cutting the specimen in small slices and placing in fixative immediately
   b handling the sections more carefully during microtomy
   c decreasing the time that the tissue is in fixative
   d increasing the paraffin infiltration time

*182 All of the following are steps in the glutaraldehyde fixation procedure for electron microscopy specimens EXCEPT:

   a initial fixation in phosphate buffered glutaraldehyde
   b rinsing with phosphate buffer following fixation
   c rinsing with gum sucrose following the buffer wash
   d postfixation in osmium tetroxide solution

*183 The BEST antibody for determining when tissue has been overfixed is:

   a S-100
   b CD20
   c vimentin
   d Cam 5.2

*184 For HER2 antibody testing, it is recommended that the fixative be:

    a acetone
    b formalin
    c Bouin
    d none

*185 Tissue antigens are irreversibly blocked by fixation in:

    a B-5
    b acetic zinc formalin
    c Bouin
    d glutaraldehyde

*186 Microscopic examination of smears stained by the Papanicolaou method show impaired nuclear staining. One possible explanation is that:

    a Gill II hematoxylin was used
    b the smears were allowed to air-dry
    c Bismarck brown was too concentrated
    d the sections were spray-fixed while wet

*187 The nuclear problem seen in this image could have been prevented by fixation that was:

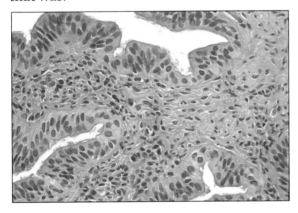

    a decreased
    b prolonged
    c immediate
    d delayed

*188 Which of the following fixatives is BEST when used at approximately neutrality?

    a glyoxal
    b formalin
    c Bouin
    d Zenker

*189 Relatively unnoted formalin pigment by light microscopy may be visualized if the microscopic slide is examined with which of the following types of microscopy?

    a transmission electron
    b dark field
    c polarizing
    d fluorescence

*190 The fixative solution has been changed, and the pathologists are not happy with the staining results given by the new method. This is probably because the stain has not been adjusted to account for the difference in:

    a penetration
    b cell shrinkage
    c fixative binding sites
    d enzyme preservation

*191 Many aqueous fixatives penetrate poorly because of:

    a enzyme activity
    b fatty cell membranes
    c conformational changes
    d pH

*192 Formalin pigment has been classified by some authors as:

    a endogenous lipidic
    b endogenous hematogenous
    c endogenous nonhematogenous
    d exogenous metallic

The following items have been identified as appropriate for both entry level histotechnicians and histotechnologists.

1 **a**	23 **a**	45 **c**	67 **d**	89 **d**	111 **b**
2 **d**	24 **c**	46 **d**	68 **b**	90 **d**	112 **b**
3 **a**	25 **d**	47 **c**	69 **d**	91 **d**	113 **b**
4 **b**	26 **c**	48 **b**	70 **c**	92 **b**	114 **d**
5 **b**	27 **d**	49 **d**	71 **b**	93 **d**	115 **b**
6 **d**	28 **c**	50 **a**	72 **b**	94 **a**	116 **b**
7 **c**	29 **a**	51 **b**	73 **a**	95 **d**	117 **a**
8 **a**	30 **a**	52 **d**	74 **b**	96 **b**	118 **d**
9 **a**	31 **c**	53 **d**	75 **b**	97 **c**	119 **c**
10 **c**	32 **b**	54 **c**	76 **c**	98 **c**	120 **c**
11 **b**	33 **d**	55 **a**	77 **c**	99 **b**	121 **c**
12 **d**	34 **d**	56 **c**	78 **d**	100 **c**	122 **a**
13 **a**	35 **c**	57 **a**	79 **b**	101 **a**	123 **c**
14 **a**	36 **d**	58 **d**	80 **c**	102 **c**	124 **a**
15 **c**	37 **b**	59 **a**	81 **a**	103 **c**	125 **d**
16 **a**	38 **d**	60 **b**	82 **b**	104 **c**	126 **d**
17 **a**	39 **b**	61 **c**	83 **b**	105 **b**	127 **c**
18 **d**	40 **d**	62 **b**	84 **b**	106 **c**	128 **c**
19 **b**	41 **b**	63 **a**	85 **a**	107 **d**	
20 **c**	42 **c**	64 **a**	86 **a**	108 **b**	
21 **d**	43 **b**	65 **d**	87 **d**	109 **b**	
22 **a**	44 **c**	66 **a**	88 **b**	110 **c**	

The following items (*) have been identified as more appropriate for entry level histotechnologists.

*129 **d**	*141 **b**	*153 **c**	*165 **d**	*177 **a**	*189 **c**
*130 **d**	*142 **c**	*154 **c**	*166 **b**	*178 **b**	*190 **c**
*131 **c**	*143 **a**	*155 **d**	*167 **d**	*179 **b**	*191 **b**
*132 **c**	*144 **a**	*156 **b**	*168 **c**	*180 **d**	*192 **b**
*133 **c**	*145 **d**	*157 **d**	*169 **c**	*181 **a**	
*134 **a**	*146 **c**	*158 **a**	*170 **c**	*182 **c**	
*135 **a**	*147 **a**	*159 **c**	*171 **c**	*183 **c**	
*136 **a**	*148 **c**	*160 **c**	*172 **d**	*184 **b**	
*137 **a**	*149 **c**	*161 **b**	*173 **b**	*185 **d**	
*138 **b**	*150 **d**	*162 **c**	*174 **d**	*186 **b**	
*139 **d**	*151 **c**	*163 **c**	*175 **c**	*187 **b**	
*140 **a**	*152 **a**	*164 **b**	*176 **c**	*188 **b**	

 ISBN 978-089189-6494   ©ASCP 2016

The following items have been identified as appropriate for both entry level histotechnicians and histotechnologists.

1   **a**   Although picric acid is considered an additive fixative, its reaction with proteins is not completely understood. [Carson & Cappellano, p17]

2   **d**   Zinc is not as toxic as mercury and has been substituted for mercury in the mercury-containing fixatives, as well as added to formaldehyde, because of the comparable, or increased, nuclear detail and increased antigenicity. [Carson & Cappellano, pp17, 22]

3   **a**   If tissue is incompletely fixed before placing in the dehydrating solution, a nuclear bubbling artifact may result. [Brown, p9; Carson & Cappellano, pp26, 28]

4   **b**   When a prolonged delay in fixation occurs, some cells may completely disappear, such as the epithelial cells in the intestinal tract. GI specimens should be opened, pinned out, and placed in fixative immediately upon receipt. [Carson & Cappellano, pp26,27]

5   **b**   Tissue for immunofluorescence studies must be unfixed and when unfixed tissue is to be held for several days or transported over a long distance, then Michel transport medium is recommended. [Carson & Cappellano, pp7,24]

6   **d**   The cupric acetate present in Hollande solution stabilizes RBC membranes, so that the lysis that occurs with Bouin solution, and other acetic acid containing fixatives, is much less. [Carson & Cappellano, p21]

7   **c**   When the microwave oven is used for fixation, irreversible morphologic damage will result if the temperature is not carefully controlled. [Carson & Cappellano, p3]

8   **a**   Hollande solution is a modification of Bouin solution, which contains acetic acid, and thus will decalcify small specimens of bone. None of the other fixatives listed are acidic. [Carson & Cappellano, p21]

9   **a**   Hollande solution contains cupric acetate, which will stabilize RBC membranes and the granules of eosinophils and endocrine cells. [Carson & Cappellano, p21]

10   **c**   Marked lysis of erythrocytes is characteristic of fixatives containing acetic acid. [Carson & Cappellano, p10]

11   **b**   Additive fixatives chemically link, or add themselves onto, the tissue and change it with this action. [Carson & Cappellano, p3; Kiernan, pp15]

12   **d**   Glutaraldehyde is a dialdehyde, and the extra aldehyde group is not involved in most crosslinking reactions; therefore, it is left free to react in any method using Schiff reagent, such as the periodic acid-Schiff (PAS) stain, for the detection of aldehydes. This leads to false positive results. [Carson & Cappellano, p14]

13   **a**   Uric acid crystals are water soluble, so can be maintained in the tissue only with a fixative solution containing no water. Absolute alcohol is recommended. [Carson & Cappellano, p7]

Answers–Fixation

Answers–Fixation

14 **a** A delay in fixation will cause improper preservation of the tissue. The nuclei may show a loss or complete disappearance of chromatin; the tissue may also show disruption of the cytoplasm, cell shrinkage, artifactual spaces around cells, or complete loss of some cells. [Carson & Cappellano, pp5, 26]

15 **c** A fixative should stabilize the tissue elements, so that the effect of any subsequent procedures, such as processing, will be minimal. [Carson & Cappellano, p2]

16 **a** Commercial formaldehyde contains about 10-14% methanol which is added to help prevent polymerization to paraformaldehyde, a highly polymeric form of formaldehyde. [Carson & Cappellano, p10]

17 **a** The cracks in the tissue and the smudgy nuclei are due to incomplete fixation. [Brown, p5; Carson & Cappellano, p26]

18 **d** Zamboni solution, glutaraldehyde, and osmium tetroxide function as fixatives for specimens for electron microscopy. Osmium tetroxide may be used either as a primary or a secondary fixative. Zamboni solution and glutaraldehyde are usually followed by osmium tetroxide to increase fat retention, and thus membrane preservation. [Carson & Cappellano, pp14, 16, 22, 25]

19 **b** Sodium borate is not a fixative. [Carson & Cappellano, pp16, 17, 23]

20 **c** Picric acid is a sufficiently strong acid to hydrolyze nuclei, so if stains for DNA (Feulgen) or RNA are anticipated, any fixative containing picric acid (Bouin, Gendre, Hollande) should be avoided. [Carson & Cappellano, p16]

21 **d** 100 mL of 70% alcohol containing 3 mL of ammonium hydroxide will remove formalin pigment when slides are placed in this solution for 30 minutes to 3 hours. [Carson & Cappellano, p25]

22 **a** Solutions of neutralized formalin prepared by storing the solution over a layer of calcium carbonate will gradually become acidic, because the pH has not been stabilized by buffering the solution. [Carson & Cappellano, p11, 13]

23 **a** When poorly fixed tissue is processed and embedded, the staining results are most often not optimum and are very difficult, if not impossible, to remedy. [Carson & Cappellano, p6]

24 **c** 300 mL of 37%-40% formaldehyde solution added to 2,700 mL of water will yield a total of 3,000 mL of a 10% formalin solution. [Carson & Cappellano, p10]

25 **d** The major use of acetic acid in fixatives is the precipitation, or coagulation, and preservation of nucleoproteins. [Carson & Cappellano, p9]

26 **c** Aldehyde fixatives are used for electron microscopy preparations because they preserve cell ultrastructure. They must be followed by secondary osmium tetroxide fixation to preserve lipids. [Carson & Cappellano, pp14, 16, 25]

27 **d** Tissue that has been fixed in a solution containing potassium dichromate will be very receptive to eosin staining. [Carson & Cappellano, pp17, 111]

28 **c** Poor penetration and excessive shrinkage will result if mercuric chloride is used alone for fixation. It is a powerful protein coagulant and enhances staining by leaving the tissues very receptive to dyes. [Carson & Cappellano, p15]

29 **a** The pigment is black acid hematin, or formalin pigment, which tends to form when the pH of the solution drops below 6.0; this may happen in unbuffered formalin solutions. The pigment may be removed by treating with saturated alcoholic picric acid. [Carson & Cappellano, p11]

30 **a** Osmium tetroxide penetrates very poorly, and so specimens should be minced to approximately 1 mm cubes for electron microscopy and cut very thin for demonstrating fat in paraffin sections. [Carson & Cappellano, pp16, 25]

31 **c** The tissue shown in this image is spleen. [Young & Lowe, p233]

32 **b** Traditionally, tissue fixed in Bouin solution is washed with 50%-70% alcohol, or 70% alcohol saturated with lithium carbonate, before processing. If excess picric acid is left in embedded tissue, the staining will deteriorate. [Carson & Cappellano, p20]

33 **d** PTAH stains are not good after formalin fixation. Zenker fixative has been used traditionally, but Bouin solution and other mordants are also effective. [Carson & Cappellano, pp179, 180]

34 **d** The problem shown in this image is nuclear bubbling. [Carson & Cappellano, pp6, 26, 28]

35 **c** Absolute ethanol will dissolve lipids, and therefore should not be used if lipid preservation is important. [Carson & Cappellano, p24, 183]

36 **d** Glutaraldehyde is a dialdehyde. The extra aldehyde group does not form crosslinks with the tissue, leaving one aldehyde group free to react in techniques depending on the demonstration of aldehydes (eg, PAS). [Carson & Cappellano, p14]

37 **b** Formaldehyde solutions become acidic by reacting with atmospheric oxygen to form formic acid; therefore, most formalin solutions require raising the pH, or preferably buffering to approximate neutrality Formic acid is undesirable because it leads to the formation of formalin pigment. [Carson & Cappellano, p11]

38 **d** In general, an increase in temperature increases the rate of fixation but also increases the rate of autolysis and diffusion of cellular elements. [Carson & Cappellano, p4]

39 **b** Carnoy solution exhibits good nuclear preservation, but lyses red blood cells, dissolves lipids, and is not recommended for the preservation and subsequent demonstration of acid-fast bacilli. [Carson & Cappellano, pp24, 216, 322]

Answers–Fixation

Answers–Fixation

40   **d**   Good preservation of tissue for light microscopy is least dependent on fixative pH, and many fixatives are quite acidic. Varying the pH from 4 to 9 apparently makes little difference in the fine structure produced by formalin fixation; however, a pigment is produced at the lower pH. The other factors listed are very important. [Carson & Cappellano, p8]

41   **b**   Formalin pigment is generally created in tissues fixed in formalin when the pH falls below 6. This pigment may be formed by any acidic fixative containing formaldehyde. [Carson & Cappellano, p11]

42   **c**   Because blood sometimes obscures important cellular detail in very bloody cytology smears, Clark solution is used to lyse the red blood cells. [Carson & Cappellano, p322]

43   **b**   Glyoxal fixatives are extremely rapid in action, and surgical specimens are fixed after only 4 to 6 hours exposure. Glyoxal forms crosslinks only under very specific conditions, lyses erythrocytes, and there may be a slight reduction in staining especially after long periods of storage. [Carson & Cappellano, p15]

44   **c**   Sections can usually be mordanted, or postfixed, in the fixative required for yielding the best staining results. [Carson & Cappellano, p7]

45   **c**   The nuclear problem seen in this image is smudgy nuclei, or the lack of a visible chromatin pattern, especially in the epithelium. [Brown, p8; Carson & Cappellano, p28]

46   **d**   Bouin solution is an excellent fixative for biopsy specimens of the gastrointestinal tract and of the endocrine system. [Carson & Cappellano, p20]

47   **c**   B-5 fixative contains mercuric chloride, sodium acetate, and 37%-40% formaldehyde. [Carson & Cappellano, p19]

48   **b**   Iodine followed by sodium thiosulfate is used for the removal of the pigment caused by mercury-containing fixatives. [Carson & Cappellano, p25]

49   **d**   Bouin solution is indicated as a mordant for trichrome stains if the tissue was not originally fixed in that solution. [Carson & Cappellano, pp20, 162, 163]

50   **a**   Decomposition of tissue by enzymatic action begins as soon as the blood supply is interrupted; therefore, the tissue should be placed in fixative solution immediately after removal. [Carson & Cappellano, pp2, 5]

51   **b**   Calcium formalin is recommended especially for the fixation and preservation of phospholipids in tissues. Phospholipids tend to take up water and extend their surface by growing outward in wormlike myelin forms; calcium ions have a dramatic effect in preventing this. [Carson & Cappellano, p12]

52   **d**   The volume of the fixative solution should be at least 15-20 greater than the volume of the tissue. [Carson & Cappellano, p5]

53   **d**   Ultrastructural preservation will be poor following fixation in 10% aqueous formalin. Formalin solutions should be buffered to neutrality and the tonicity adjusted for use as a fixative for electron microscopy. [Carson & Cappellano, p11]

54   **c**   Glyoxal is the smallest dialdehyde. [Carson & Cappellano, p15]

55 **a** Zinc-formalin fixatives will give poor ultrastructural preservation. Zinc is a protein coagulant and the fixatives used for ultrastructural studies are noncoagulants. [Carson & Cappellano, pp4, 25]

56 **c** Zamboni refers to a buffered picric acid-formaldehyde solution that may be used as a general purpose fixative. It allows secondary fixation with osmium tetroxide and preserves the morphologic characteristics accurately; therefore, it is useful for both light and electron microscopy. [Carson & Cappellano, p22, 25]

57 **a** The problem in this section could have been prevented by slicing the specimen upon receipt, placing it in fixative and allowing plenty of time for complete fixation. [Brown, p4; Carson & Cappellano, pp5, 6, 26]

58 **d** Stains for fat are done on frozen sections, and the preferred fixative is neutral buffered formalin. [Carson & Cappellano, p183]

59 **a** Cytology smears should be fixed within 1-2 seconds, or an air-drying artifact will most likely occur. [Carson & Cappellano, p315]

60 **b** After osmium tetroxide fixation, cell cytoplasm has little affinity for the anionic (acid, eg, eosin) dyes, but will readily accept cationic (basic) dyes. [Carson & Cappellano, p16, 111]

61 **c** The breakdown of tissue due to enzyme activity is called autolysis. Putrefaction is caused by bacterial action, polymerization is a chemical reaction in which 2 or more small molecules join together to form a larger molecule, and osmosis refers to diffusion through a semipermeable membrane. [Carson & Cappellano, pp2, 8]

62 **b** Urate crystals found in gouty tophi are water soluble; therefore, an aqueous based fixative cannot be used; absolute alcohol is the fixative of choice. [Carson & Cappellano, p7, 24]

63 **a** A good fixative for routine use should make the tissue more permeable to fluids, so that all subsequent processes occur readily. [Carson & Cappellano, p3]

64 **a** Chromate-containing fixatives should be washed with water before processing because the dehydrating alcohol can cause an insoluble pigment to form. [Carson & Cappellano, p17]

65 **d** The pH, time and temperature of fixation, and the concentration and purity of the reagents all play an important role in the proper preservation of the ultrastructure. The type of tissue is not important. [Carson & Cappellano, pp4-8]

66 **a** Formic acid in formalin leads to the formation of black acid hematin, or formalin pigment. [Carson & Cappellano, p11]

67 **d** Carnoy solution contains chloroform, glacial acetic acid, and absolute alcohol. [Carson & Cappellano, p24]

Answers–Fixation

68   **b**   A primary chromate fixative is necessary for the preservation of chromaffin granules. The demonstration of these granules are used for the diagnosis of pheochromocytoma. [Carson & Cappellano, p7]

69   **d**   2% to 3% glutaraldehyde is an excellent fixative for the preservation of tissue ultrastructure. Secondary fixation with osmium tetroxide is necessary to chemically react with and preserve the lipids before processing for EM. [Carson & Cappellano, pp14, 25]

70   **c**   Slow penetration of tissue is an undesirable fixative characteristic. [Carson & Cappellano, p7, 8]

71   **b**   Some of the epithelium is gone in this section, indicating that there was a slight delay in fixation. GI specimens should be opened, pinned out, and placed in fixative as soon after interruption of the blood supply as possible. [Carson & Cappellano, pp4, 5, 26]

72   **b**   Bouin solution does not contain absolute alcohol. [Carson & Cappellano, p20]

73   **a**   Coagulant fixatives establish a meshlike network in tissue that allows solutions to readily penetrate or gain entry into the interior of the tissue. [Carson & Cappellano, p3]

74   **b**   Tissue breakdown by bacterial action is known as putrefaction. [Carson & Cappellano, p2]

75   **b**   When ultrastructural preservation is the main purpose of fixation, the solution should be buffered to a pH of 7.2-7.4; this is a physiologic pH, or approximately the pH of tissue fluid. [Carson & Cappellano, p8]

76   **c**   Mercuric salts will produce a brownish-black pigment in tissues. [Carson & Cappellano, p15]

77   **c**   The best solution for long term storage of tissue is 70% alcohol; this preserves both routine and immunohistochemical staining properties. [Carson & Cappellano, p8]

78   **d**   Ethyl alcohol is a precipitant fixative solution that is used primarily for the fixation of water soluble substances, such as glycogen and urate crystals. It is a nonadditive fixative that has no effect on tissue basophilia, and it shrinks and overhardens tissue. [Carson & Cappellano, pp4, 24]

79   **b**   Nuclear bubbling is most often the result of placing the incompletely fixed tissue in the dehydrating solutions. [Brown, p9; Carson & Cappellano, p6]

80   **c**   Formalin solutions should be buffered to a pH of 6.8-7.4 in order to prevent the formation of formalin pigment; this pigment usually occurs if the pH drops below 6.0. [Carson & Cappellano, p11]

81   **a**   Specimens may remain in 10% neutral buffered formalin indefinitely, and this is not true of the other fixatives listed; so if the date of processing is not definite, then formalin is the best choice. [Carson & Cappellano, p7]

82   **b**   Placing a specimen in water will cause the cells to take up water and swell and rupture as a result. Placing tissue in any hypotonic solution can have this effect. [Carson & Cappellano, p8]

83   **b**   If the temperature of the microwave oven is allowed to exceed 68°C, the tissue will show pyknotic, overstained nuclei. [Carson & Cappellano, p3]

84   **b**   An alcoholic solution saturated with picric acid is commonly used to remove formalin pigment; melanin pigment is usually bleached with an oxidizing agent; hemosiderin, or iron pigment, is usually demonstrated with the Prussian blue reaction;, and mercury pigment is removed by iodine. [Carson & Cappellano, pp24, 25, 251]

85   **a**   Formaldehyde is a reducing agent, and will reduce some of the chemicals present in Helly solution. This results in the solution turning dark and turbid. [Carson & Cappellano, p21]

86   **a**   Monobasic and dibasic sodium phosphates are commonly used to buffer formaldehyde solutions for routine use. [Carson & Cappellano, p13]

87   **d**   The preferred fixative for the trichrome procedure shown in this image is Bouin solution. [Carson & Cappellano, pp7, 162]

88   **b**   Zamboni fixative is a buffered formaldehyde-picric acid that is a good dual purpose fixative; that is, it is good for both light and electron microscopy. [Carson & Cappellano, p22]

89   **d**   Methanol is the best fixative for blood smears. [Carson & Cappellano, p24]

90   **d**   Osmium tetroxide vaporizes readily and the vapor itself readily fixes the nasal mucosa or the conjunctiva; contact with the vapor must be avoided, and thus it must be used under a chemical hood. [Carson & Cappellano, p16]

91   **d**   Calcium formalin is recommended for phospholipid preservation for any histochemical studies. [Carson & Cappellano, p12]

92   **b**   Formalin ammonium bromide is recommended for the fixation of tissue for staining with the Cajal method for astrocyte demonstration. [Carson & Cappellano, p12-13]

93   **d**   Hollande solution is a modification of Bouin solution. [Carson & Cappellano, p21]

94   **a**   Tissue fixed in B-5 solution must be treated for the removal of the mercury pigment; B-5 solution contains mercuric chloride, sodium acetate, and formaldehyde. [Carson & Cappellano, p19-20]

95   **d**   Acetone is recommended for frozen sections of brain tissue to be stained for a diagnosis of rabies. [Carson & Cappellano, p23]

96   **b**   Fresh, unfixed tissue can be stored safely for a short time by wrapping it in saline-dampened gauze (excess saline squeezed out), and placing it on ice or in the refrigerator. It should never be placed in physiologic saline. [Carson & Cappellano, p24]

97   **c**   The smudgy nuclei, or lack of chromatin definition, seen in this image is attributed to incomplete fixation of the tissue. [Brown, p5; Carson & Cappellano, p26, 28]

98   **c**   Bouin solution is the best fixative for connective tissue stains; if tissue is fixed in formalin, the sections should be mordanted in Bouin solution before staining with trichrome procedures. Bouin solution is excellent for preserving structure with soft and delicate textures, lyses red cells, and has good penetration. [Carson & Cappellano, pp7,20,162-163]

99   **b**   The heat generated by microwaves will physically fix tissue. [Carson & Cappellano, p2]

100   **c**   Alcohol or Carnoy solution is preferred if Congo red staining for amyloid is to be done, although other fixatives may be used. [Carson & Cappellano, p154]

101   **a**   Spirochetes are usually stained with silver methods, and 10% formalin is the preferred fixative for most silver stains. Mercurial and chromate fixatives should be avoided. [Carson & Cappellano, pp21, 235]

102   **c**   Zinc salts are frequently added to formalin solutions to preserve antigenicity, or immunoreactivity. [Carson & Cappellano, p17]

103   **c**   *Helicobacter pylori* organisms will not stain satisfactorily after glyoxal fixation. [Carson & Cappellano, p15]

104   **c**   Acetone has been used historically for the preservation and subsequent demonstration of the enzymes acid and alkaline phosphatase. [Carson & Cappellano, p23]

105   **b**   Acetic acid is sometimes added to fixative solutions to counteract the shrinkage caused by another component. [Carson & Cappellano, p10]

106   **c**   Formaldehyde crosslinks proteins by forming methylene bridges that link protein chains together. [Bancroft & Gamble, p56; Carson & Cappellano, p3]

107   **d**   Trichrome stains are most commonly used for the distinction between collagen and muscle, and Bouin solution is the best fixative for trichrome procedures. [Carson & Cappellano, pp7, 162-163]

108   **b**   The picric acid in Bouin solution is strong enough to hydrolyze nucleic acid, and should not be used if stains for DNA or RNA are anticipated. [Carson & Cappellano, p15]

109   **b**   Acetic acid is sometimes used in fixative solutions to counteract the shrinking effect of another component. [Carson & Cappellano, p10]

110   **c**   Since 10% formalin is a 1:10 dilution of 37–40% formaldehyde, 10% formalin solutions actually contain 3.7- 4% formaldehyde and are equivalent to a 4% paraformaldehyde solution. [Carson & Cappellano, p10]

111   **b**   Since 95% alcohol produces the shrinkage and sharpness of the nuclear membrane resulting in the nuclear detail characteristic of cytologic preparations, other alcohols must be substituted in the strength that will result in the same nuclear detail. 80% isopropyl alcohol and 100% methyl alcohol cause the same shrinkage as 95% ethyl alcohol, and yield the same nuclear detail. [Carson & Cappellano, p317]

112 **b** Osmium tetroxide chemically combines with lipids, making them insoluble for subsequent dehydrating and clearing solutions. [Carson & Cappellano, p16]

113 **b** Acetic acid lyses red blood cells and any fixative containing acetic acid will show this lysis. [Carson & Cappellano, p10]

114 **d** Formalin pigment is likely to occur, especially in bloody areas, if the pH of the solution drops below 6.0; therefore, it should be buffered to neutrality. [Carson & Cappellano, p11]

115 **b** Osmium tetroxide penetrates very poorly, so sections should be cut very thin for fixation for paraffin embedding. [Carson & Cappellano, p16]

116 **b** Mercuric salts penetrate poorly, and will produce shrinkage or will allow shrinkage in the subsequent processing steps. [Carson & Cappellano, p15]

117 **a** Picric acid causes extreme shrinkage or allows extreme shrinkage to occur in subsequent processing steps; therefore, it is combined with acetic acid in Bouin solution to counteract this shrinkage. [Carson & Cappellano, p10 ,20]

118 **d** Of the fixatives listed, only B-5 will preserve erythrocytes; all other contain acetic acid which will lyse erythrocytes. [Carson & Cappellano, pp10, 19]

119 **c** The pigment is most likely a result of acidic formalin fixation and can be removed with an alcoholic solution of picric acid. The only other possible pigment is that formed by mercuric salts, and it is removed by iodine (not listed). [Carson & Cappellano, pp11, 25]

120 **c** Alcohol causes extreme shrinkage and hardening of tissue, and should be used only when a non-aqueous fixative is needed. [Carson & Cappellano, p24]

121 **c** Only formalin should be used as a fixative if sections are to be stained by the Warthin-Starry technique. [Bancroft & Gamble, p67; Carson & Cappellano, p234]

122 **a** The pigment has occurred in a bloody area; therefore, it is most likely formalin pigment. [Carson & Cappellano, p11]

123 **c** The tissue is small intestine. [Carson & Cappellano, p27]

124 **a** The fixative of choice for preserving fat is formalin; then it can be demonstrated on a frozen section. However, it will be removed during routine processing. [Carson & Cappellano, p10]

125 **d** Picric acid hydrolyzes nucleic acids, so the sections cannot be used for the demonstration of DN A and RNA. Picric acid shrinks tissue, increases eosin uptake, and leaves tissue soft. [Carson & Cappellano, p16]

126 **d** The primary purpose of fixation is to stabilize proteins. [Carson & Cappellano, p2]

127 **c** Clark solution is used to lyse erythrocytes in bloody cytology specimens because of its content of acetic acid. [Carson & Cappellano, pp10, 24, 322]

128 **c** Epithelium is the tissue component most affected by the problem shown in the image. [Carson & Cappellano, p5; Young & Lowe, p168]

Answers–Fixation

The following items (*) have been identified as more appropriate for entry level histotechnologists.

*129 **d** Glutaraldehyde is a dialdehyde, and one aldehyde group is left free during fixation; therefore, it is free to react with the Schiff reagent used in the PAS technique giving nonspecific staining. [Carson & Cappellano, p14]

*130 **d** Urate crystals will be dissolved if the specimen is fixed in an aqueous-based fixative solution, and will give negative results when stained or polarized. [Carson & Cappellano, p7]

*131 **c** Formaldehyde reacts primarily with the NH_2 group by forming crosslinks. [Bancroft & Gamble, p56; Carson & Cappellano, p10]

*132 **c** Phosphates can cause precipitation of zinc, so tissue fixed in zinc-formalin solutions should be washed before transferring to phosphate-buffered formalin. [Carson & Cappellano, p23]

*133 **c** Osmium fixes fats, and cell membranes have phospholipids as a major component; therefore, cell membranes will become electron-dense after fixation in osmium tetroxide. [Carson & Cappellano, p16]

*134 **a** Michel medium is a transport medium used for unfixed tissue that is to be held for several days or transported over a long distance; it is frequently used for the transportation of kidney biopsies for immunofluorescence. [Carson & Cappellano, p24]

*135 **a** Specimens from the gastrointestinal tract should be opened as soon as possible after interruption of the blood supply, pinned out, and covered with fixative. This will prevent any autolysis of the epithelium. [Brown, p4; Carson & Cappellano, p6, 26]

*136 **a** A change in fixative solution is likely to change the isoelectric point of the cytoplasmic proteins, and difference in eosin uptake will be noted. [Carson & Cappellano, p3]

*137 **a** Enzymes continue to act even after the blood supply is interrupted and this will cause autolysis; the amount of autolysis that occurs is determined by the delay in fixation. The GI tract will show the loss of epithelium and if the delay is significant, the lamina propria is also affected. [Carson & Cappellano, p2]

*138 **b** The problem seen in this image is most often seen in tissue that was taken postmortem. [Carson & Cappellano, pp2, 5-6]

*139 **d** If tissue has been fixed for enzyme histochemical studies, it may be stored in gum sucrose solution (30% sucrose solution containing 1% gum acacia) at 4°C for several weeks. [Carson & Cappellano, p296]

*140 **a** Before freezing tissue that has been transported in Michel transport medium, the tissue should be washed with mild agitation in 3 8-minute changes of phosphate-buffered saline containing 10% sucrose. [Carson & Cappellano, p24]

*141 **b**   Body fluids have an osmolality of about 340 mOsm, so isotonic solution would have an equivalent mOsm. [Carson & Cappellano, p8]

*142 **c**   Overheating in the microwave oven will give pyknotic nuclei and marked distortion of architecture; carefully controlling the temperature is a must with microwave fixation. [Carson & Cappellano, p3]

*143 **a**   Picric acid is fairly acidic and preferably is washed out with alcohol to which lithium carbonate has been added as a neutralizer before processing. If picric acid remains in the tissue when it is embedded, the staining characteristics will change, and eventually become extremely poor. [Carson & Cappellano, p17]

*144 **a**   The most common cause of nuclear bubbling is incomplete fixation before the tissue is placed in alcohol, so extending the time of fixation to ensure adequate fixation should prevent nuclear bubbling. [Brown, p8; Carson & Cappellano, p6, 26, 28]

*145 **d**   Specimens for electron microscopy cannot be left in osmium tetroxide for more than 2-4 hours. [Carson & Cappellano, p25]

*146 **c**   All of the fixatives listed are used primarily for electron microscopy, and only Zamboni PAF is stable at room temperature. [Carson & Cappellano, p14, 16, 22]

*147 **a**   Paraformaldehyde must be heated to 60°C and made slightly alkaline to depolymerize, or dissociate, it to formaldehyde. [Carson & Cappellano, p10]

*148 **c**   For electron microscopy, tissue fixed in glutaraldehyde must be postfixed in osmium tetroxide. [Carson & Cappellano, p25]

*149 **c**   Displaced mitochondrial membranes are a good indicator of poor fixation of electron microscopy specimens. [Carson & Cappellano, p25]

*150 **d**   70% alcohol containing ammonium, sodium, or potassium hydroxide may be used to remove formalin pigment. [Carson & Cappellano, p25]

*151 **c**   Fixatives that contain aldehydes mask antigenic sites and hamper immunohistochemical localization of antigens. [Carson & Cappellano, p266; Kiernan, p514]

*152 **a**   Smudgy, or muddy, nuclei are the result of incomplete fixation. [Brown, p5; Carson & Cappellano, p26]

*153 **c**   Osmium tetroxide cannot be used in immunoelectron microscopy because it has a harsh, deleterious effect on the antigenicity of the tissue. [Bancroft & Gamble, p605]

*154 **c**   Orth solution does not contain mercuric chloride, but does contain formaldehyde, potassium dichromate, and acetic acid. [Carson & Cappellano, p22]

*155 **d**   Of the fixatives listed, buffered formalin should be chosen for fixation. Acid-fast stains are not satisfactory after Carnoy fixation, and Zenker solution and B-5 solutions require long periods of fixation and postfixation washing and/or pigment removal. [Carson & Cappellano, pp19, 21, 216]

*156 **b**   Microwaves create instantaneous heat, and heat is a method of physical fixation. [Carson & Cappellano, p2]

*157 **d**   B-5 solution contains mercury, and mercury must be removed from sections prior to staining by treatment with iodine. [Carson & Cappellano, p19-20, 25]

*158 **a**   The sections must have been fixed in Zenker fluid, which contains chromium trioxide, and not washed carefully before placing the tissue in alcohol. The alcohol will reduce the chromium and forms an insoluble pigment in the tissue. [Carson & Cappellano, p17]

*159 **c**   The nonimmunohistochemical stain needed is a PTAH, which requires fixation in a solution other than formalin; therefore, the section will need to be mordanted in another fixative before staining with the PTAH technique. [Carson & Cappellano, pp178-180]

*160 **c**   Formalin pigment can be seen in this section; it could have been prevented by ensuring that the formalin used for fixation was buffered to approximate neutrality. [Brown, p8; Carson & Cappellano, p11]

*161 **b**   Fixation of tissue for electron microscopy with osmium tetroxide should be brief, preferably one hour or less. Specimens should never be left longer than 4 hours. [Carson & Cappellano, p25]

*162 **c**   Formaldehyde is a reducing agent and will reduce the chromium present in Helly solution, turning it turbid; therefore, the formaldehyde must be added just before use. [Carson & Cappellano, p21]

*163 **c**   The acetic acid will lyse erythrocytes, and the acidic formalin will result in the formation of a brown crystalline pigment known as formalin pigment. [Carson & Cappellano, pp10, 11]

*164 **b**   The precipitate is most likely paraformaldehyde, a polymer of formaldehyde, and it should be disregarded. [Carson & Cappellano, p10]

*165 **d**   Acetone can be used for the fixation of cell surface antigens. It would dissolve the fat in myelin sheaths and phospholipids, and would inactivate oxidoreductases. [Carson & Cappellano, pp23, 184, 209, 309

*166 **b**   Formalin that is not buffered will gradually become acidic upon standing, and if used for fixation, it will produce formalin pigment in tissues. Formalin solution should be buffered and the pH will change very little over time. [Carson & Cappellano, p11]

*167 **d**   The stain used in the diagnosis of rhabdomyosarcoma is the PTAH, and this stain requires fixation in a solution other than formalin; therefore, tissue fixed in formalin requires mordanting in another fixative. [Carson & Cappellano, pp178, 179]

*168 **c**   This section of small intestine did not have immediate contact with the fixative solution and much of the surface epithelium has been lost. [Carson & Cappellano, p27]

*169 **c**   A gouty tophus is a formed by urate crystals, and these crystals are water soluble; therefore, a non-aqueous fixative should be used. Absolute alcohol is the fixative of choice. [Carson & Cappellano, p7]

*170 **c**   To ensure adequate fixation the tissue should be place in a minimum of 240 mL of solution. [Carson & Cappellano, p4]

*171 **c**   Acetone overhardens tissue dramatically, but preserves glycogen, and some enzymes. It is frequently used on froze sections of tissue to be stained for cell surface antigens by immunohistochemical techniques. [Carson & Cappellano, p23]

*172 **d**   Tissue fixed in Bouin solution will not give good ultrastructural preservation, and is unsatisfactory for electron microscopic studies. [Carson & Cappellano, p20]

*173 **b**   Immunohistochemical staining is the best technique for use in the diagnosis of malignant melanoma. [Carson & Cappellano, p290]

*174 **d**   The tissue has been improperly fixed for the demonstration of urate crystals because urates are water soluble. [Carson & Cappellano, p7]

*175 **c**   Clark solution does not contain chloroform, whereas Carnoy solution does. [Carson & Cappellano, p24]

*176 **c**   Osmium tetroxide will not preserve chromaffin granules, a chromate containing fixative (eg, Orth solution) should be used for this purpose. [Carson & Cappellano, p7]

*177 **a**   An aqueous fixative must be used if lipids are to be preserved. [Carson & Cappellano, pp10, 16, 24, 184]

*178 **b**   New regulations state that fixation of tissue for HER2 testing should be no less than 6 hours and no more than 48 hours. [Carson & Cappellano, p266]

*179 **b**   Tissues that undergo the most rapid autolysis are those that are rich in enzymes, such as liver, pancreas, and brain. [Carson & Cappellano, p2]

*180 **d**   Pap smears that have been fixed with a spray fixative must be placed in 95% alcohol for approximately 15 minutes before staining, or the nuclei will appear foggy and lack detail. [Carson & Cappellano, p317, 327]

*181 **a**   The problem shown can be prevented in the future by slicing the spleen in small slices (bread-loafing) and placing the slices in fixative immediately upon receipt. [Carson & Cappellano, p26]

*182 **c**   Fixation in phosphate buffered glutaraldehyde for electron microscopy is followed by a phosphate buffer wash and postfixation in osmium tetroxide; no gum sucrose wash is used. [Carson & Cappellano, pp14, 25]

*183 **c**   Vimentin is most often the antibody used to detect overfixation of specimens for immunohistochemistry. [Carson & Cappellano, p267]

*184 **b**   New regulations recommend formalin fixation of breast tissue for HER2 antibody testing. [Carson & Cappellano, pp266]

*185 **d**   Fixation in glutaraldehyde will irreversibly block tissue antigens. [Carson & Cappellano, p14]

*186 **b**   Cytology smears that are allowed to air dry will show a loss of chromatin patterns and nuclear swelling, and eosinophilic cytoplasm and a loss of cytoplasmic density. [Carson & Cappellano, p317]

Answers–Fixation

*187 b   Fixation was not complete, and should have been prolonged; this resulted in muddy nuclei. [Brown, p5; Carson & Cappellano, p26, 28]

*188 b   All of the fixatives except formalin are acidic; formalin should be approximately neutral to prevent the formation of formalin pigment. Glyoxal is preferably used at pH 4.0. [Brown, p8; Carson & Cappellano, p11, 15, 20, 21; Kiernan, p31]

*189 c   Formalin pigment is birefringent, and if present, will show up with polarization. [Brown, p8; Carson & Cappellano, p11]

*190 c   Different fixatives will bind to different tissue sites, dramatically affecting the uptake of eosin especially. When fixatives are changed, the staining procedure should be evaluated and possibly changed. [Brown, p1; Carson & Cappellano, pp3, 10, 22, 119]

*191 b   Unless there are channels for fixatives to traverse, the solution must pass through one cell to get to the next, and the fatty cell membrane will impede the passage of aqueous fixatives. [Brown, p1]

*192 b   Because it may occur intracellularly and is formed by the reaction with heme, formalin pigment was considered by Vacca to be endogenous hematogenous. [Carson & Cappellano, pp11, 242]

Processing

The following items have been identified as appropriate for both entry level histotechnicians and histotechnologists.

1   During microtomy, it is noted that many of the tissues are very hard and shrunken. Of the following, the most likely explanation for this problem is that the:

    a infiltrating paraffin is too hot
    b processing reagents need changing
    c pH of the fixative was incorrect
    d clearing agent is contaminated with water

2   Decalcification of small specimens can be achieved by fixation in:

    a neutral buffered formalin
    b Zenker solution
    c glutaraldehyde
    d Zamboni solution

3   A major disadvantage of aliphatic clearing agents is that they:

    a are incompatible with some mounting media
    b have a very high penetration rate
    c harden tissue excessively
    d are highly toxic

4   Which of the following is MOST likely to cause sensitization with prolonged use?

    a cedarwood oil
    b xylene
    c aliphatic hydrocarbons
    d limonene

5   To speed up the laboratory's processing of all surgical tissues, the temperature of all fixation, dehydration, and clearing steps has been set at 45°C. This will most likely result in:

    a excellent sections of all tissue
    b very soft uterine scrapings
    c microchatter
    d sections that will not stain with eosin

6   Limonene functions as a/an:

    a clearing agent only
    b dehydrating agent only
    c universal solvent
    d infiltrating medium

7   One advantage of aliphatic hydrocarbons is that they:

    a have a high tolerance for water
    b are miscible with all mounting media
    c are low in toxicity and sensitization
    d are adaptable to various processing methods

8   A disadvantage of using heat at all stations of the tissue processor is that it will:

    a harden some tissues
    b lengthen processing time
    c shorten the processor lifespan
    d cause too much reagent evaporation

9   Dehydration refers to the removal of:

    a alcohol
    b paraffin
    c water
    d xylene

10   Which decalcification method may cause heat damage to the specimen?

    a acid
    b chelation
    c electrolytic
    d ion exchange

11   Which of the following clearing agents is NOT flammable?

    a benzene
    b chloroform
    c toluene
    d xylene

12   Which of the following groups of reagents may be used for dehydration?

    a ethanol, limonene, and tetrahydrofuran
    b methanol, ethanol, and limonene
    c dioxane, methanol, and toluene
    d dioxane, methanol, and ethanol

13   The decalcifying agent EDTA is NOT an excellent choice when bone specimens will:

    a be stained with immunohistochemical procedures
    b be allowed long exposure to the decal reagent
    c have enzymes demonstrated in the bone
    d require diagnosis within 48 hours

14   A clearing agent must be miscible with:

    a dehydrants and infiltrating media
    b fixatives and dehydrants
    c fixatives and infiltrating media
    d universal solvents

15   Which of the following is a chelating agent used for decalcification?

    a ethylenediaminetetraacetic acid
    b hydrochloric acid
    c trichloracetic acid
    d phenol

16   The alcohols on the tissue processor should be changed on a regular basis because:

    a the alcohols become saturated with bile from gall bladder specimens, which can be absorbed by other tissues
    b too great a concentration of formalin in the alcohols can create a potentially explosive situation
    c Gram negative organisms can start growing in alcohol left too long on the tissue processor
    d the alcohols absorb moisture and become dilute

17   After completion of decalcification, the specimen should be:

    a placed in acetone
    b rinsed with 70% alcohol
    c transferred to fixative
    d washed in water

18   Which of the processing schedules shown below should be used to process fixed routine surgical tissue?

schedule A		schedule B		schedule C	
formol-alcohol	2 hours	80% alcohol	20 minutes	80% alcohol	8 hours
95% alcohol	1 hour	80% alcohol	20 minutes	95% alcohol	4 hours
95% alcohol	1 hour	95% alcohol	20 minutes	95% alcohol	4 hours
absolute alcohol	1 hour	95% alcohol	20 minutes	absolute alcohol	4 hours
absolute alcohol	1 hour	absolute alcohol	20 minutes	absolute alcohol	4 hours
xylene	1 hour	absolute alcohol	20 minutes	chloroform	1 hour
xylene	1 hour	absolute alcohol	20 minutes	chloroform	1 hour
paraffin	1 hour	xylene	20 minutes	chloroform	1 hour
paraffin	1 hour	xylene	20 minutes	paraffin	2 hours
paraffin	1 hour	paraffin	20 minutes	paraffin	2 hours
paraffin	20 minutes	paraffin	20 minutes	paraffin	2 hours

  a schedule A
  b schedule B
  c schedule C
  d none of the above is adequate

19   Ethanol functions as a(n):

  a dehydrating agent
  b clearing agent
  c universal solvent
  d infiltrating medium

20   Which of the processing schedules shown below should be used to process a fixed needle biopsy of the liver?

schedule A		schedule B		schedule C	
formol-alcohol	2 hours	80% alcohol	20 minutes	80% alcohol	8 hours
95% alcohol	1 hour	80% alcohol	20 minutes	95% alcohol	4 hours
95% alcohol	1 hour	95% alcohol	20 minutes	95% alcohol	4 hours
absolute alcohol	1 hour	95% alcohol	20 minutes	absolute alcohol	4 hours
absolute alcohol	1 hour	absolute alcohol	20 minutes	absolute alcohol	4 hours
xylene	1 hour	absolute alcohol	20 minutes	chloroform	1 hour
xylene	1 hour	absolute alcohol	20 minutes	chloroform	1 hour
paraffin	1 hour	xylene	20 minutes	chloroform	1 hour
paraffin	1 hour	xylene	20 minutes	paraffin	2 hours
paraffin	1 hour	paraffin	20 minutes	paraffin	2 hours
paraffin	20 minutes	paraffin	20 minutes	paraffin	2 hours

    a schedule A
    b schedule B
    c schedule C
    d none of the above is adequate

21   Butyl alcohol is recommended as a dehydrant for:

    a blood smears
    b brain tissue
    c plant tissue
    d spleen

22   The processing step that assures alcohol is removed from the tissue is:

    a fixation
    b dehydration
    c clearing
    d infiltration

23   Dehydrating tissues in graded alcohols of increasing concentrations is superior to using absolute alcohol ONLY because it will:

    a cause less distortion of the tissue
    b be less harmful to the tissue processor
    c not harden tissue over a long period
    d remove the fixative faster

24   For best support during microtomy, decalcified bone specimens which are processed to paraffin wax should be embedded in:

    a both agar and paraffin
    b "hard" paraffin
    c "soft" paraffin
    d celloidin

25   The BEST method of preparing tissue for enzyme demonstration is:

    a agar embedding
    b celloidin embedding
    c paraffin embedding
    d unfixed frozen sections

26   Glycol methacrylate functions as a(n):

    a dehydrating agent only
    b clearing agent only
    c universal solvent
    d infiltrating medium

27   Fat remains in the tissue following infiltration with:

    a Carbowax
    b celloidin
    c paraffin
    d glycol methacrylate

28   Methanol functions as a(n):

    a dehydrating agent only
    b clearing agent only
    c universal solvent
    d infiltrating medium

29   The most effective method for rapidly freezing tissue is using:

    a aerosol sprays
    b dry ice
    c gaseous carbon dioxide
    d liquid nitrogen/isopentane

30   The amount of time a specimen needs to remain in decalcifying solution is NOT influenced by the:

    a bone density
    b processing schedule
    c solution strength
    d solution temperature

31   When tissues have been fixed in Carnoy fluid, into which processing solution should they be placed first?

    a formalin
    b molten wax
    c 95% or 100% alcohol
    d xylene

32 Tissue must be dehydrated before placing it in:

a agar
b Carbowax
c epoxy resin
d gelatin

33 In order to process tissue faster, which of the following could be done easily and still yield good results?

a add agitation to each step
b remove vacuum from each step
c increase heat to 70°C in alcohols
d infiltrate with softer wax

34 The ideal thickness of specimens to be decalcified is:

a 1 to 2 mm
b 3 to 4 mm
c 6 to 7 mm
d 9 to 10 mm

35 Paraffin processing is contraindicated for the subsequent demonstration of:

a enzymes
b mucins
c nuclei
d proteins

36 Which of the following reagents is miscible with water, alcohol, hydrocarbons, and paraffin?

a acetone
b cedarwood oil
c dioxane
d xylene

37 Reprocessing tissue may lead to false negative immunohistochemical staining results, due to:

a alcohol fixation
b incomplete dehydration
c repeated xylene exposure
d repeated exposure to heated paraffin

38 The LEAST desirable method to check for decalcification endpoint is:

a electrolysis
b physical
c radiologic
d chemical tests

39   Prolonged dehydration in higher grades of alcohol will render a specimen:

   a hard
   b macerated
   c porous
   d toxic

40   For adequate clearing in xylene during routine processing, tissue should have a maximum thickness of:

   a 1 to 2 mm
   b 3 to 4 mm
   c 5 to 6 mm
   d 7 to 8 mm

41   The purpose of using a hydrometer in the histopathology laboratory is to:

   a assure the temperature of the laboratory is comfortable
   b determine the percentage of alcohols used in processing
   c check urine specific gravity before urinalysis
   d determine the pH of reagents

42   Processing of delicate tissues (eg, embryonic tissues) should be started in what concentration of alcohol?

   a 30%
   b 50%
   c 70%
   d 90%

43   The hazy blue nuclear staining results seen in the image below are most commonly seen when:

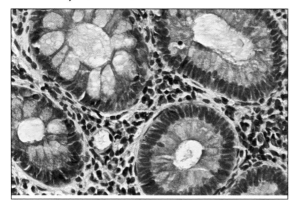

   a Celestine blue is used in place of hematoxylin
   b improper use of heat on the tissue processor
   c overstaining with Schiff reagent
   d fixation in Bouin solution

44 The effect of overdecalcification is most noticeable in the staining of:

    a nuclei
    b cytoplasm
    c erythrocytes
    d bone spicules

45 Which of the following is considered the BEST dehydrant?

    a acetone
    b ethanol
    c isopropanol
    d methanol

46 All of the following are methods for checking the completeness of decalcification EXCEPT:

    a chemical
    b electrolytic
    c mechanical
    d radiographic

47 Acid solutions soften bone tissue by removing which of the following salts?

    a calcium
    b lithium
    c potassium
    d sodium

48 The clearing reagent must be miscible with:

    a fixative and paraffin
    b fixative and dehydrant
    c dehydrant and paraffin
    d paraffin and water

49 If the clearing agent is cloudy, it may be contaminated with:

    a absolute alcohol
    b bacteria
    c water
    d yeast

50 Dioxane functions as a(n):

    a dehydrating agent only
    b clearing agent only
    c universal solvent
    d infiltrating medium

51 Which of the following gases is released during decalcification?

   a ammonia
   b carbon dioxide
   c nitrous oxide
   d oxygen

52 Evaluate the embedding of the block in the image below. Select the correct assessment.

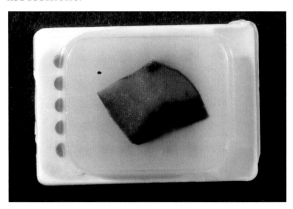

   a tissue was appropriately embedded
   b wax was allowed to cool too slowly
   c embedding mold was too large for the tissues
   d tissue was not pressed to the bottom of the mold evenly

53 The artifact seen in the center of the embedded tissue seen here is caused by:

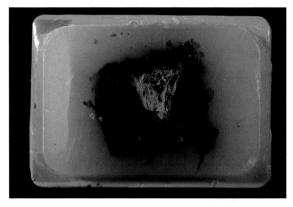

   a excess exposure to xylene
   b fixation in alcohol-containing fixative
   c insufficient dehydration
   d incorrect orientation

ISBN 978-089189-6494   ©ASCP 2016

54 The overall pink-orange coloration of the embedded uterine specimen seen in the image below is due to:

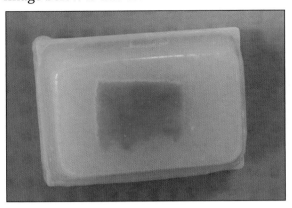

   a blood remaining in the tissue
   b fixation in Bouin solution
   c processing wax needs to be changed
   d eosin was added to processing alcohols

55 The time needed for infiltration of paraffin into a tissue specimen is dependent upon all of the following EXCEPT the:

   a fixative used
   b thickness of the specimen
   c tissue type
   d use of vacuum

56 Xylene functions as a(n):

   a dehydrating agent
   b clearing agent
   c universal solvent
   d infiltrating medium

57 Which one of the following methods of determining the endpoint of decalcification may introduce artifacts to the tissue?

   a suspension
   b physical
   c radiographic
   d chemical

58 Which of the following can be used to hold small tissue fragments or friable tissues in place for paraffin processing?

   a Carbowax
   b agar
   c paraffin
   d methacrylate

59   In the image below, what is the most likely cause of the staining results on this
      bone marrow specimen?

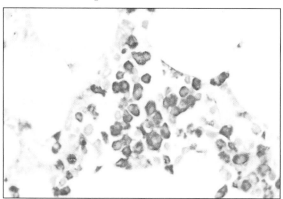

   a underdecalcification
   b overdecalcification
   c improper dehydration
   d prolonged fixation

60   Decalcification occurs with all of the following methods EXCEPT:

   a simple acid
   b radiographic
   c chelation
   d ion exchange

61   Which of the following is miscible with hydrocarbons?

   a agar
   b Carbowax
   c gelatin
   d paraffin

62   The process of saturating tissue with the medium that will be used for embedding
      is called:

   a clearing
   b dehydration
   c fixation
   d infiltration

63   Toluene functions as a(n):

   a dehydrating agent only
   b clearing agent only
   c universal solvent
   d infiltrating medium

64   Of the reagents listed below, the BEST substitute for ethanol for processing tissues is:

     a   dioxane
     b   butanol
     c   isopropanol
     d   methanol

65   Refer to the schedule shown below. If processing is started at 8:00 AM Monday, at what time on Tuesday will the tissue be ready to embed?

schedule

80% alcohol 8 hours
95% alcohol 4 hours
95% alcohol 4 hours
absolute alcohol 4 hours
absolute alcohol 4 hours
chloroform 1 hour
chloroform 1 hour
chloroform 1 hour
paraffin 2 hours
paraffin 2 hours
paraffin 2 hours (in vacuum)

     a   4:00 PM
     b   5:00 PM
     c   6:00 PM
     d   7:00 PM

66   What is the most likely cause of the artifact seen in this image?

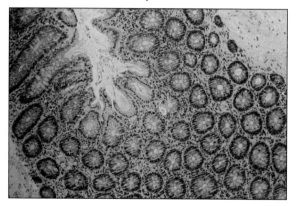

     a   incomplete fixation
     b   overdehydration during processing
     c   overheating before staining
     d   prolonged fixation

67   Which of the following must one do when using an essential oil as a clearing agent?

   a avoid the use of ethyl alcohol
   b remove the oil with xylene
   c avoid exposure to heat
   d avoid lengthy exposure

68   Freezing tissues slowly prior to sectioning will most likely:

   a make sectioning difficult
   b yield sections showing tissue disruption
   c require a change in the knife clearance angle
   d preserve antigenic sites

69   After H&E staining, a decalcified tissue shows some areas of very dark purple staining. The most likely explanation is:

   a prolonged decalcification in strong acid
   b bone was not left in decalcification solution long enough
   c wax was not completely removed from section before staining
   d tissue was initially fixed in formalin

70   Determining the endpoint of decalcification is very important because:

   a calcium remaining in the tissue interferes with staining
   b underdecalcification causes processing problems
   c overdecalcification results in destruction of cell structure
   d prolonged acid treatment inhibits good fixation

71   Paraffin with a melting point of 55°C is used for impregnation and embedding. The temperature of the paraffin containers should be regulated at approximately:

   a 50°C
   b 55°C
   c 58°C
   d 62°C

72   For complete infiltration of tissue with paraffin, the time needed depends on the:

   a melting point of the paraffin
   b thickness and texture of the tissue
   c choice of dehydrating agent
   d the fixative used

73   The step in tissue processing that must be completed before dehydration is:

   a infiltration
   b antigen retrieval
   c clearing
   d fixation

74   All of the following are criteria for choosing a suitable clearing agent for use on the tissue processor, EXCEPT:

   a cost
   b rapid removal of fixative
   c removal by paraffin
   d flammability

75   Paraffin belongs to this class of chemicals:

   a low weight alkanes
   b long chain hydrocarbons
   c hydroxyls
   d amines

76   For BEST results, before decalcification in acids, a buffered formalin fixed specimen should be:

   a washed with water to remove phosphates
   b placed in Helly fluid to counteract the formalin
   c washed in water to reverse incomplete fixation
   d washed in ammonia water to raise the pH

77   When EDTA is used as a decalcifier, the recommended pH of the solution is:

   a 3.0 - 4.0
   b 6.0 - 6.5
   c 7.0 - 7.4
   d 8.6 - 9.0

78   Of the following, which describes when a bone does NOT have to be fixed before decalcification?

   a specimen is a fresh bone marrow
   b nitric acid is used as the decalcifier and acts as a fixative
   c specimen is a femoral head section
   d decalcifier is combined with fixative in one solution

79   A well fixed, properly decalcified specimen will show all of the following, EXCEPT:

   a preservation of nuclear detail
   b retention of calcium in the tissue
   c differential staining of nuclei and cytoplasm
   d good tissue morphology

80   Although benzene is rarely used as a clearing agent, one advantage is that it:

   a evaporates rapidly from paraffin, so waxes don't need to be changed on processor
   b can be disposed of in the municipal water supply
   c has no evidence of toxicity
   d slow acting, so its penetration can be monitored easily

81 Of the chemical reagents used for decalcification, which one is slower acting than others?

    a hydrochloric
    b nitric
    c formic
    d EDTA

82 In order to pour decalcification acids down the drain, they must be:

    a less than 1% in concentration
    b more than pH 11
    c treated with 10% acetic acid
    d neutralized with 1% sodium bicarbonate

83 When a lab uses tetrahydrofuran in tissue processing, the type of tissue specimen that will most likely show distortion is:

    a breast reduction
    b colon resection
    c lung biopsy
    d gall bladder

84 When tissue is fixed in a formaldehyde primary fixative and then placed directly in hydrochloric acid for decalcification, what is an expected outcome?

    a the carbon dioxide that is released smells like motor oil
    b a carcinogen can be chemically formed
    c the bone will decalcify much slower than when specimen is washed
    d any calcium salts will sink to the bottom of the container

85 Which of the following acid decalcification methods requires LESS frequent changing of the solution?

    a ion exchange
    b hydrochloric acid used alone
    c heated hydrochloric acid
    d EDTA

86   In the image below, the artifact seen in the H&E stained frozen section of skeletal muscle could have been caused by:

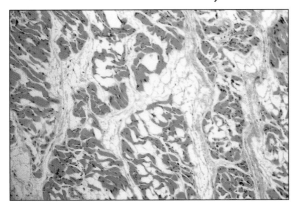

   a xylene was used as a clearing agent
   b section was not fixed before staining
   c biopsy was frozen in the cryostat at –20°C
   d tissue was not oriented properly before cutting

87   Ethyl alcohols used in tissue processing may be made unfit for human consumption by the commercial addition of:

   a eosin
   b xylene
   c methanol
   d water

88   When surface decalcification is employed during microtomy, the following steps are recommended:

   a face the block and then treat with decalcification solution
   b place un-faced block into EDTA for 30 to 60 minutes
   c hold a gauze soaked in ammonia on the block face for 5 minutes
   d float the ribbon on a water bath filled with 5% nitric acid

89   The schedule for monitoring decalcification completeness should be:

   a every 3 to 4 hours when EDTA is used
   b once a day, for any decalcification solution
   c once every 2 days when any 5% acid solution is used
   d depends on strength of decal solution used

90   Microwave processing is most useful for which of the following specimen types?

   a mastectomy
   b transplant biopsy
   c colon resection
   d appendix

91 When employing microwave processing, the tissue sample should be:

   a up to 4 mm thick
   b processed in a household microwave oven
   c heated above 84°C
   d fixed before processing

92 The major benefit of microwave processing is:

   a decreased time for completion
   b increased reagent use
   c no fixation needed
   d temperatures up to 80°C are achieved

93 During paraffin processing, how many changes of paraffin wax are recommended for adequate infiltration?

   a 1
   b 2
   c 3
   d 4

94 When a fixed liver biopsy is received in the laboratory for rapid processing, it is recommended that:

   a processing starts in 100% alcohol
   b xylene steps last minimum of 3 hours
   c paraffin temperature be raised to 70°C
   d fixative solutions be skipped

95 To assist the embedder in identifying small and colorless tissue samples after processing, it is recommended that:

   a the same person who grosses the tissue must also embed it
   b the processing cassette be marked to indicate the specimen is small
   c a small amount of eosin be added to the last dehydrating reagent
   d colored paraffin be added for infiltration

96 Dehydration during tissue processing occurs by repeated dilution or by the:

   a hydrophilic property of alcohol
   b dessicant's action in the chamber
   c addition of phloxine to the xylene
   d action of the clearant

97 When a block of under-decalcified bone is being cut and a section cannot be obtained, the BEST course of action would be to:

   a chill the block with freeze-spray
   b increase the clearance angle of the knife
   c melt the block down and reprocess
   d place the faced surface in 5% HCl

98   One purpose of the additives that are in some paraffin wax is to:

    a assist orientation of tissues
    b increase hardness
    c retard solidification
    d decrease condensation

99   The method most commonly used in cytology preparation of a sparsely cellular nongynecologic fluid specimen is:

    a needle aspiration
    b crush method
    c cytocentrifugation
    d homogenization

100 In order to process tissue faster, which of the following could be done easily and still yield results?

    a add vacuum to each reagent step
    b increase heat to 70°C at each station
    c use butanol in place of ethanol
    d infiltrate with a harder wax

101 How often should the processing reagents be changed on the processor?

    a every day
    b once a week
    c depends on the amount of use
    d once a month

102 When small biopsy and large tissue specimens are processed together with a processing schedule that will adequately process the larger specimens, what is the likely outcome for the biopsy specimens?

    a fat in the specimens will be soft and mushy
    b over-hardening and dryness
    c incomplete fixation
    d improved nuclear preservation

103 To assure adequate and appropriate tissue processing, in which processing step should heat be applied?

    a dehydration
    b clearing
    c infiltration
    d all of the above

104 Resins used for electron microscopy processing:

    a are cut with a rotary microtome
    b harden by polymerization
    c require formalin fixation
    d harden by crystallization

The following items (*) have been identified as more appropriate for entry level histotechnologists.

*105 A technologist in the electron microscopy laboratory has developed dermatitis. This problem can most likely be prevented in the future by ensuring that:

   a a chemical hood is used for processing
   b the secondary fixation step is eliminated
   c another resin is selected for embedding
   d protective gear is worn during processing

*106 Smudgy nuclei and variations in nuclear staining are noted on routinely processed, formalin fixed colon biopsy specimens. One cause of these problems could be:

   a overfixation
   b incomplete dehydration
   c poor choice of fixative
   d prolonged clearing

*107 Processed tissue that was fixed in zinc-formalin is very hard and brittle. The stained sections show microscopic chatter. This problem might be corrected in the future by:

   a leaving the tissue in the fixative for less than 4 hours
   b treating the tissue for removal of pigment
   c placing the tissue in a buffer solution after fixation
   d selecting a better schedule for processing

*108 A technologist in the electron microscopy laboratory has developed dermatitis. This is probably because of exposure to:

   a osmium tetroxide
   b absolute ethanol
   c epoxy resin
   d the electron beam

*109 When placed in a solution whose refractive index is similar to the refractive index of tissue proteins, tissue becomes:

   a fragile
   b hard
   c small
   d translucent

*110 Microscopic review of H&E stained sections of a colon biopsy show very uneven staining of the tissue and poor nuclear detail. Of the following, the most likely cause is that the:

   a paraffin block was cooled too slowly
   b tissue remained in alcohol too long
   c pH of the fixative was incorrect
   d clearing agent is contaminated with water

*111 Xylene, toluene, and benzene belong to what chemical class?

    a hydrocarbon
    b ketone
    c phenol
    d sterol

*112 To help maintain morphology in formalin fixed tissue prior to freezing, fixed tissue may be placed in a solution of:

    a gum mastic
    b saline
    c sucrose
    d talc

*113 Consider the viscosity (in centipoises) at 20°C of the various solutions given below. Which of the solutions would clear most quickly?

    a benzene (0.65)
    b butanol (2.95)
    c toluene (0.59)
    d xylene (0.7)

*114 The penetration of any solution into tissue is increased as which of the following is increased?

    a molecular size of the solution
    b temperature of the solution
    c viscosity of the solution
    d specific gravity of the solution

*115 To BEST demonstrate muscle enzymes, which freezing method should be used?

    a cryostat freezer plate
    b dry ice
    c liquid nitrogen
    d isopentane, prechilled to –150° C

*116 Refer to the schedule shown below. If the processing run starts at 12 noon, at what time will it be appropriate to add a specimen being processed for the subsequent demonstration of urate crystals?

schedule
80% alcohol 20 minutes
80% alcohol 20 minutes
95% alcohol 20 minutes
95% alcohol 20 minutes
absolute alcohol 20 minutes
absolute alcohol 20 minutes
absolute alcohol 20 minutes
xylene 20 minutes
xylene 20 minutes
paraffin 20 minutes
paraffin 20 minutes
paraffin 2 hours

  a 12 noon
  b 1:00 PM
  c 1:40 PM
  d 3:30 PM

*117 Polyethylene glycol is employed as the embedding medium for the preservation of:

  a enzymes
  b urate crystals
  c lipids
  d keratin

*118 Increasing the pressure inside the tissue processing chamber provides which of these advantages?

  a reagents stay cooler, thereby preventing heat damage to tissues
  b boiling point of solvents is increased
  c flow of fluids into tissue spaces is improved
  d dehydration is slowed, thereby decreasing over-dehydration

*119 Consider the viscosity (in centipoises) at 20°C of various solutions given below. Which of the solutions would dehydrate most quickly?

  a acetone (.3)
  b ethanol (1.2)
  c isopropanol (2.5)
  d methanol (.6)

*120 Consider the viscosity (in centipoises) at 20°C of the various solutions given below. Which would dehydrate most slowly?

    a acetone (.3)
    b ethanol (1.2)
    c isopropanol (2.5)
    d methanol (.6)

*121 Consider the viscosity (in centipoises) at 20°C of various solutions given below. Which of the following solutions would clear most slowly?

    a acetone (.3)
    b benzene (.65)
    c toluene (.59)
    d xylene (.7)

*122 The results seen in the acid-decalcified, H&E stained bone marrow in the image below could have been caused by failing to:

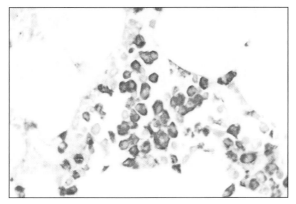

    a wash fixative out of specimen before decalcification
    b wash specimen after decalcification
    c store decalcification solution in the refrigerator
    d orient the section properly at embedding

*123 When processing with water soluble wax, tissue is fixed, washed with water, and:

    a dehydrated with 95% and absolute alcohols, cleared with xylene, and then infiltrated
    b dehydrated with 95% alcohol and then infiltrated
    c dehydrated and cleared with a universal solvent and then infiltrated
    d infiltrated only

*124 Which of the following should be selected when tissue must be embedded in a medium that will tolerate a small amount of water?

    a glycol methacrylate
    b celloidin
    c Epon
    d paraffin

*125 If a laboratory ran out of ethanol, which of the following dehydrants might be available and suitable for emergency use?

a dioxane
b tetrahydrofuran
c isopropanol
d butanol

*126 The practice of "double embedding" generally employs these 2 types of compounds:

a resin and agar
b paraffin and resin
c agar and paraffin wax
d paraffin wax and methacrylate

*127 High resolution light microscopy is needed on a lymph node biopsy. To achieve the BEST results, the specimen should be processed for embedding in:

a water soluble wax
b celloidin
c glycol methacrylate
d microcrystalline wax

*128 A section of kidney is fixed in phosphate-buffered formalin and then routinely processed with 95% alcohol, absolute alcohol, xylene, and paraffin. When sectioned, many vertical knife lines are noted in the sections, and these lines remain in the same area of the tissue even when the knife is moved. This is most likely due to:

a precipitated phosphates in the tissue
b defects in the knife edge
c excessive dehydration of the tissue
d poor fixation

*129 Carbowax has a major disadvantage of:

a dissolving during flotation
b being a lengthy processing method
c making tissues brittle for sectioning
d causing cell shrinkage

*130 Paraffin infiltration at 70°C would:

a make tissue easier to section
b preserve lipids better
c shorten infiltration time by 50%
d denature tissue antigens

 ISBN 978-089189-6494   ©ASCP 2016

*131 An oil red O stain has been requested on a friable specimen that must be embedded for sectioning. The embedding medium that should be used is:

   a plastic
   b paraffin
   c water soluble wax
   d celloidin

*132 Microwave processing generally uses which of the following reagents?

   a formalin instead of alcohols
   b isopropyl alcohol for dehydration and clearing
   c ethyl alcohol and xylene
   d saline for fixation and dehydration

*133 While performing the daily temperature check of the embedding center paraffin reservoir, it is noted that the temperature is 12° above the melting point of paraffin. The most appropriate action is to:

   a drain and replace the paraffin
   b check the thermostat setting
   c recheck the temperature in 24 hours
   d do nothing; the temperature is acceptable

*134 A method of decalcification is needed for research bone specimens on which subsequent oxidative enzyme stains are essential. Which of the following decalcifying methods should be selected?

   a electrolytic
   b ion exchange
   c chelating agents
   d simple acid

*135 A research project requires a sectioning procedure with the following specifications:

    - contact with water must be avoided in sectioning
    - there must be minimum distortion of tissue
    - fat stains can be done on the sections
    - procedure may require several hours

To which of the following processing techniques do these specifications refer?

   a resin
   b celloidin
   c paraffin
   d water soluble wax

*136 In the electrolytic method of decalcification, the specimen to be decalcified is attached to the anode. The reason for this is that:

   a calcium ions will become neutralized at this site
   b proteins are more readily neutralized at this site
   c insoluble calcium salts will form on the anode
   d calcium ions will migrate to the cathode

*137 According to the graph of paraffin bath temperatures shown below, how many days of the week may reveal problems in microtomy? The melting point of the paraffin is 56°C-58°C.

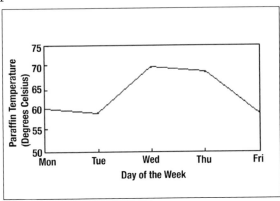

   a none
   b 1
   c 2
   d 3

*138 In order to maintain the BEST tissue morphology in tissue samples to be decalcified, it is imperative that:

   a tissue is fixed prior to decalcification
   b staining times are shortened to counteract increased basophilia
   c tissue is treated with zinc salts after decalcification
   d electrolytic method is performed on specimens

Using the processing schedules below, answer the next 3 questions (139, 140, & 141).

	schedule A	schedule B	schedule C
buffered formalin 1	4 hours 15 minutes	10 minutes	skip
buffered formalin 2	30 minutes	10 minutes	skip
95% alcohol 1	45 minutes	5 minutes	skip
95% alcohol 2	45 minutes	5 minutes	10 minutes
100% alcohol 1	45 minutes	5 minutes	skip
100% alcohol 2	45 minutes	skip	10 minutes
100% alcohol 3	1 hour	10 minutes	10 minutes
xylene 1	45 minutes	10 minutes	skip
xylene 2	45 minutes	skip	10 minutes
xylene 3	1 hour	10 minutes	10 minutes
paraffin 1	1 hour	10 minutes	10 minutes
paraffin 2	1 hour	15 minutes	10 minutes

                ISBN 978-089189-6494   ©ASCP 2016

*139 The processor schedule A would be WORST suited for which specimen population?

a gastric biopsies
b decalcified bone
c colon resections
d large breast mass

*140 Look at processing schedule A. If the processor was scheduled to have reagents rotated or "bumped up," which reagents would be dumped from their containers?

a 95% 1, 100% 2, and xylene 1
b 95% 1, 100% 1, and xylene 1
c 95% 2, 100% 3, and xylene 3
d 95% 1 & 2, 100% 3, and xylene 1 & 2

*141 Which type of tissue specimen would be processed adequately when processed using schedule C?

a Eyeball
b fatty breast
c fixed needle biopsy
d cervical cone

*142 After H&E staining, it is noted that tissue processed overnight all lack chromatin definition in the nuclei, and there is variable nuclear staining properties. What is a likely cause of this staining result?

a inadequate fixation
b prolonged dehydration
c water remained in tissues during infiltration
d sections grossed too thick

*143 In order to assure that very small tissue pieces or cellular specimens are not lost during processing, it may be required to place the specimen in which of the following before placing it on the tissue processor?

a liquid agar and allowed to solidify
b methacrylate resin and polymerized
c nitrocellulose and hardened
d chloroform and allowed to evaporate

*144 The appropriate method used for processing a body fluid with spontaneous clots is to:

a squeeze out excess liquid from clot and wrap clot in lens paper
b make a cell block using the agar method
c make a cell block using the albumin method
d filter the fluid and scrape cells off the filter paper

*145 The pathologist is concerned because there are too many occurrences of the artifact shown in this image. The most likely source of the problem is:

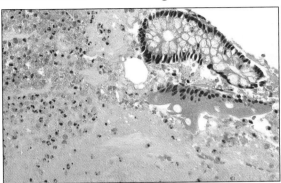

   a tissue carryover in the staining reagents
   b contaminated embedding paraffin
   c specimen packed too tightly in the cassette
   d forceps not cleaned between specimens

*146 In which of the following areas would the supervisor expect to have to monitor the personnel most closely to determine the source of the artifact seen in the image above?

   a microtomy
   b staining
   c embedding
   d processing

*147 There have been problems with tissue autofluorescence in fluorescence in situ hybridization (FISH) procedures. One possible cause is the use of:

   a reagent alcohol for dehydration
   b eosin in the dehydrant
   c paraffin embedded tissue
   d a commercially made probe

*148 To avoid tissue autofluorescence, a good colorant for the processor dehydrating solution is:

   a erythrocin
   b methylene blue
   c eosin
   d phloxin

The following items have been identified as appropriate for both entry level histotechnicians and histotechnologists.

1 a	19 a	37 d	55 a	73 d	91 d
2 b	20 b	38 b	56 b	74 b	92 a
3 a	21 c	39 a	57 b	75 b	93 c
4 d	22 c	40 b	58 b	76 a	94 d
5 c	23 a	41 b	59 b	77 c	95 c
6 a	24 b	42 a	60 b	78 d	96 a
7 c	25 d	43 b	61 d	79 b	97 d
8 a	26 d	44 a	62 d	80 a	98 b
9 c	27 a	45 b	63 b	81 d	99 c
10 c	28 a	46 b	64 c	82 d	100 a
11 b	29 d	47 a	65 b	83 c	101 c
12 d	30 b	48 c	66 b	84 b	102 b
13 d	31 c	49 c	67 b	85 a	103 c
14 a	32 c	50 c	68 b	86 c	104 b
15 a	33 a	51 b	69 b	87 c	
16 d	34 b	52 d	70 c	88 a	
17 d	35 a	53 c	71 c	89 d	
18 a	36 c	54 d	72 b	90 b	

The following items (*) have been identified as more appropriate for entry level histotechnologists.

*105 d	*113 c	*121 d	*129 a	*137 c	145 d
*106 b	*114 b	*122 b	*130 d	*138 a	146 c
*107 d	*115 d	*123 d	*131 c	*139 a	147 b
*108 c	*116 c	*124 a	*132 b	*140 b	148 b
*109 d	*117 c	*125 c	*133 b	*141 c	
*110 d	*118 c	*126 c	*134 c	*142 c	
*111 a	*119 a	*127 c	*135 d	*143 a	
*112 c	*120 c	*128 a	*136 d	*144 a	

©ASCP 2016   ISBN 978-089189-6494

The following items have been identified as appropriate for both entry level histotechnicians and histotechnologists.

1 **a** When tissue is processed in paraffin wax that is more than 2°C to 4°C above the melting point, the tissue becomes hard and shrunken. [Carson & Cappellano, p38]

2 **b** Because Zenker contains acetic acid, it can decalcify needle biopsies of bone marrow. [Carson & Cappellano, p21]

3 **a** Aliphatic xylene substitutes are incompatible with mounting media, because most mounting media contain toluene or xylene. [Carson & Cappellano, p36]

4 **d** Limonene causes sensitization and allergic reactions in some individuals. [Carson & Cappellano, p35]

5 **c** Excess heat during processing, especially in dehydration and clearing, can lead to removal of bound water and results in microchatter during microtomy. [Carson & Cappellano, pp32, 37, 41]

6 **a** Limonene is used as a xylene substitute, making it a clearing agent. [Carson & Cappellano, p35]

7 **c** Aliphatic hydrocarbons are less toxic and lead to less sensitization than aromatic hydrocarbons used as clearing agents. [Carson & Cappellano, p36]

8 **a** When heat is used in all stations of the processor (especially dehydration and clearing), the tissues become hard. [Carson & Cappellano, p38]

9 **c** The term "dehydration" means removal of water. [Carson & Cappellano, p33]

10 **c** Electrolytic methods of decalcification may cause damage to the specimen because of the heat generated by the method. [Carson & Cappellano, p47]

11 **b** Chloroform is not flammable or combustible, but when heated, it may form a toxic gas. [Carson & Cappellano, p35]

12 **d** The 3 reagents listed are all used for dehydration. Dioxane also may be used as a universal solvent. [Carson & Cappellano, pp33-35]

13 **d** The decalcifying reagent EDTA does not damage tissues, and immunohistochemical and enzyme reactions can be performed after its use. It is very slow in action, and a 24-hour time frame is not sufficient time for EDTA to decalcify bone. [Carson & Cappellano, p48]

14 **a** Clearing agents must be miscible with the reagents used both directly before and after it. [Carson & Cappellano, p34]

15 **a** EDTA is the chelating agent employed in decalcification. [Carson & Cappellano, p48]

16 **d** Because alcohols remove water from tissues, they become more diluted with water and less effective at further dehydration of tissues. [Carson & Cappellano, p32]

17 **d** In order to stop the activity of acid decalcifying solutions, it is necessary to wash the tissue. Continued acid activity in the tissue will lead to over-decalcification and impaired staining of the tissue. [Carson & Cappellano, p48]

ISBN 978-089189-6494 ©ASCP 2016

18   **a**   Schedule A allows time for routine tissue specimens to have complete fixation, dehydration, clearing and infiltration. [Carson & Cappellano, p38]

19   **a**   Ethanol is an alcohol, and a very good dehydrating agent. [Carson & Cappellano, p33]

20   **b**   Fixed small biopsies will be adequately processed using Schedule B. The longer processing times will lead to over-dehydration and hardening of the biopsy. [Carson & Cappellano, p38]

21   **c**   One of the main uses of butanol is for dehydrating plant material. [Carson & Cappellano, p33]

22   **c**   Clearing removes alcohol from tissues prior to infiltration with wax. [Carson & Cappellano, p34]

23   **a**   Tissue shrinkage is minimized when graded alcohols are used instead of going directly from an aqueous fixative to 100% alcohol. [Carson & Cappellano, p33]

24   **b**   Decalcified bone sectioning is made easier after infiltration and embedding in a harder paraffin wax. [Bancroft & Gamble, p343; Carson & Cappellano, p37]

25   **d**   In order to prevent a decrease in enzymatic activity, processing that requires heat is avoided. [Carson & Cappellano, p296]

26   **d**   Glycol methacrylate is an infiltration medium that is converted to a solid by polymerization. [Carson & Cappellano, p40]

27   **a**   Because Carbowax processing does not require the use of solvents that would dissolve lipids, the fat remains in tissue. [Carson & Cappellano, p39]

28   **a**   Methanol is one of the alcohols that is used for dehydration, although it is rarely used alone for tissue dehydration. [Carson & Cappellano, p33]

29   **d**   In order to prevent the formation of freeze artifact in tissue, rapid freezing with isopentane cooled in liquid nitrogen is the preferred freezing technique. [Carson & Cappellano, p50]

30   **b**   Bone density, decal solution strength and solution temperature all influence the time necessary for decalcification to occur. Processing schedules have no impact on decalcification. [Carson & Cappellano, pp47-49]

31   **c**   When tissue has been fixed in a nonaqueous fixative such as Carnoy, it should be placed directly in 95% or 100% alcohol for processing. [Bancroft & Gamble, p83; Carson & Cappellano, p24]

32   **c**   Tissue to be infiltrated and embedded in epoxy resins must be completely dehydrated prior to placing the tissue in resin. [Carson & Cappellano, p40]

33   **a**   Agitation of the processing solutions aids in reagents' flow thru the tissues, leading to decreased time necessary for good processing. [Bancroft & Gamble, p84]

34   **b**   For adequate penetration of decalcification fluids into and through calcified specimens, they should be cut at 3-4 mm. [Bancroft & Gamble, p338]

35   **a**   The heat used in paraffin processing will destroy enzymatic activity. [Carson & Cappellano, p296]

Answers–Processing

36 **c** Dioxane is used as a universal solvent, which indicates that it is miscible with water, alcohols, hydrocarbons, and paraffins. [Carson & Cappellano, p34]

37 **d** Antigens are altered by high temperatures, and the repeated exposure to hot wax during reprocessing may alter the epitope sites such that false negative results are seen. [Carson & Cappellano, p267]

38 **b** Physical methods of checking the endpoint of decalcification may introduce artifacts (such as holes or breaks) to the tissue. [Carson & Cappellano, p48]

39 **a** Tissues become hard when left in high grades of alcohol for long periods of time. [Carson & Cappellano, p33]

40 **b** For adequate penetration of processing fluids into and through specimens, they should be cut at 3 - 4 mm. [Bancroft & Gamble, p83]

41 **b** Hydrometers measure specific gravity and may also be calibrated to read the percentage of alcohol, and are used in histopathology for checking alcohols for the correct strength. [Carson & Cappellano, p38]

42 **a** Delicate tissues may be distorted when placed in higher concentrations of alcohol, due to the diffusion currents that cross membranes and cause distortion. [Bancroft & Gamble, p85]

43 **b** The hazy blue nuclear staining is the result of the use of heat in the tissue processor alcohol and xylene steps. [Carson & Cappellano, p37]

44 **a** Over-exposure to decalcification acids decreases nuclear basophilia. [Carson & Cappellano, p50]

45 **b** Of all the alcohols, ethanol is considered the best dehydrant. [Carson & Cappellano, p33]

46 **b** Electrolytic procedures are not used for checking the endpoint of decalcification. [Carson & Cappellano, p48]

47 **a** Acids remove calcium from bone so that it is soft enough to be cut in paraffin. [Carson & Cappellano, p47]

48 **c** The clearing agent must be miscible with reagents directly before and after it; therefore, it must be miscible with the dehydrating fluid and wax. [Carson & Cappellano, p34]

49 **c** Hydrocarbons used in clearing tissues turn cloudy in the presence of water. [Carson & Cappellano, p34]

50 **c** Dioxane can be used for both dehydration and clearing of tissues. [Carson & Cappellano, p34]

51 **b** Carbon dioxide is formed during decalcification with acids. [Carson & Cappellano, p47]

52 **d** The tissue was not evenly pressed to the bottom of the mold during embedding, resulting in tissue at various depths in the block. This often leads to incomplete sections taken at microtomy. [Carson & Cappellano, p46]

53 **c** The center of this block is not completely fixed and/or processed, so it is still soft. It will not section properly, and should be reprocessed. [Carson & Cappellano, p45]

ISBN 978-089189-6494   ©ASCP 2016

54 **d**   The orange-pink color of this tissue is due to the addition of eosin or phloxine to the processing alcohols, which ensures that small colorless biopsies are more easily identified at embedding, but all tissues take up the coloration. [Carson & Cappellano, p32]

55 **a**   The fixative used on a specimen will have no impact on the time needed for paraffin infiltration. [Carson & Cappellano, pp37-38]

56 **b**   Xylene is the most commonly used hydrocarbon clearing agent. [Carson & Cappellano, p34]

57 **b**   Physical manipulation of a specimen for determining the endpoint of decalcification may introduce artifacts such as holes or breaks in the bone. [Carson & Cappellano, p48]

58 **b**   Tissue fragments are placed in liquid agar and it is allowed to solidify before processing to paraffin block, ensuring that all pieces of tissue are captured for embedding and cutting. [Carson & Cappellano, p41]

59 **b**   When bone marrow is left in decalcification acids longer than necessary to remove calcium, the nuclear basophilia is compromised. [Carson & Cappellano, p48, 50]

60 **b**   Radiography is a method used for determining the endpoint of decalcification, not as a method of decalcification. [Carson & Cappellano, p48]

61 **d**   Paraffin is the only reagent listed that is miscible with hydrocarbons such as xylene. The other reagents listed are all water soluble. [Carson & Cappellano, pp37, 40-41]

62 **d**   Infiltration with wax is necessary for proper embedding of tissue in wax. [Carson & Cappellano, pp36-37]

63 **b**   Toluene, although not frequently used, is a hydrocarbon used as a clearing agent. [Carson & Cappellano, pp34-35]

64 **c**   Isopropanol is a good substitute for ethanol for dehydration during processing, but not for use in staining procedures. [Carson & Cappellano, p33]

65 **b**   By counting the time in all the processing steps, 5 PM on Tuesday is when the tissues will be ready to embed. [Carson & Cappellano, p38]

66 **b**   Too much drying from over-dehydration during processing will cause microchatter at microtomy. [Carson & Cappellano, p41]

67 **b**   When essential oils are used as clearing agents, it is necessary to remove the oil with a hydrocarbon prior to paraffin infiltration. [Carson & Cappellano, p35]

68 **b**   When tissue is frozen slowly, it is likely to show disruption in morphology caused by large ice crystals. This is especially evident in skeletal muscle biopsies. [Carson & Cappellano, p50]

69 **b**   Calcium left in tissue will stain dark purple with hematoxylin. [Carson & Cappellano, p49]

70 **c**   When calcified tissue is left in acid decalcifiers for a prolonged time, the cellular morphology is destroyed. [Carson & Cappellano, p47, 50]

71 **c**   The paraffin should not exceed temperatures 2 - 4°C above its melting point, as paraffin that is too hot will overharden tissues. [Carson & Cappellano, p37]

Answers–Processing

72   **b**   Complete infiltration depends on complete replacement of clearing agent from the tissue, and the time necessary for that process will be increased in thick and/or dense tissues; time necessary will be decreased for thin and/or less dense tissue samples. [Carson & Cappellano, p36-37]

73   **d**   When tissue is not completely fixed before dehydration, fixation in alcohol occurs and leads to increased eosinophilia at the center of the tissue. [Bancroft & Gamble, p83]

74   **b**   Clearing agents do not remove fixatives, as they are used after alcohol and before wax. The others are criteria that should be considered. [Carson & Cappellano, p34]

75   **b**   Paraffin wax is an inert mixture of hydrocarbons produced from petroleum processing. [Bancroft & Gamble, p87]

76   **a**   When phosphate salts are left in tissue samples, they may counteract the action of acid decalcifiers in the tissue. [Kiernan, p47]

77   **c**   The optimum pH of EDTA when used as a decalcifying agent is 7.0 - 7.4. [Bancroft & Gamble, p340]

78   **d**   Some proprietary decalcification fluids contain both fixative and acid, and tissues do not have to be separately fixed before being placed in the solution. [Brown, p9]

79   **b**   Decalcified tissue should not have calcium in the tissue; others are desirable aspects of specimens. [Brown, p9]

80   **a**   Benzene is very volatile, and evaporates from paraffin at its melting point; therefore, the wax stays clean of the clearing agent. [Carson & Cappellano, p35]

81   **d**   EDTA is very slow acting as a decalcifier, making its use easily controlled. [Carson & Cappellano, p48]

82   **d**   Acids used as decalcifiers should be neutralized with 1% sodium bicarbonate before flushing down the drain. [Carson & Cappellano, p48]

83   **c**   Tetrahydrofuran, as a universal solvent, causes diffusion currents that can harm delicate tissue morphology. [Carson & Cappellano, p34]

84   **b**   The carcinogen, bis-chloromethyl ether, can be formed by a reaction between formaldehyde and hydrochloric acid. [Carson & Cappellano, p47]

85   **a**   Ammonium ions from the resin used in ion exchange decalcification are exchanged for calcium, thus keeping the acid free from calcium ions. [Carson & Cappellano, p47]

86   **c**   When tissue is frozen slowly, at −20°C, large artifactual holes are often seen as a result of large ice crystals. [Carson & Cappellano, p50]

87   **c**   The addition of methanol, and sometimes isopropanol, makes ethanol unfit for consumption, thus making it non-taxable. [Carson & Cappellano, p33]

88   **a**   Before surface decalcification, the surface wax on the face of the block must be trimmed away to expose the tissue needing calcium removal. [Carson & Cappellano, p49]

89 **d** If a strong, fast acting decalcifier is used, the time it takes for decalcifying specimens will be shorter in length. If a weaker acid is used, the time required will be longer. [Bancroft & Gamble, p340; Carson & Cappellano, p47]

90 **b** Biopsy specimens are small and process well in the time and solutions utilized in microwave processing. [Carson & Cappellano, p39]

91 **d** If tissue is not well fixed prior to microwave processing, fixation will be completed by the alcohol, which will lead to morphologic changes different from the laboratory's routine. [Carson & Cappellano, p39]

92 **a** The major benefit of microwave processing is the reduction in time it affords. [Carson & Cappellano, p39]

93 **c** 3 changes of paraffin are recommended. [Carson & Cappellano, p38]

94 **d** The fixation steps can be skipped if the biopsy is already well fixed. [Carson & Cappellano, p38]

95 **c** Adding eosin to the last dehydrating alcohol gives color to small and colorless tissues, making identification of them easier for the embedder. [Carson & Cappellano, p32]

96 **a** Alcohol attracts water molecules, and in this manner it helps draw water out of tissues during dehydration on the processor. [Carson & Cappellano, p32]

97 **d** Tissue that has been under-decalcified may be soaked in acid to remove calcium from the surface of the block. [Carson & Cappellano, p49]

98 **b** The addition of plastics to paraffin increase hardness and support for hard and dense tissue. [Carson & Cappellano, p37]

99 **c** Cytocentrifugation allows essentially all the cells in a sparsely cellular fluid specimen to be deposited onto a slide, while the fluid is absorbed away onto a filter paper. [Carson & Cappellano, p321]

100 **a** Vacuum increases the rate of infiltration of processing fluids, thus decreasing the time necessary to complete the steps in processing. [Carson & Cappellano, p38]

101 **c** Each laboratory should establish its own schedule for changing processing reagents, based on the number of cassettes processed. [Carson & Cappellano, p38]

102 **b** When small biopsy specimens are processed on a schedule that is long enough to adequately process larger tissue samples, the small tissues will become hard and dry. [Carson & Cappellano, p37]

103 **c** Heat should be applied to the paraffins only, as heating other processing reagents will generally result in hard and brittle tissues. [Carson & Cappellano, p37]

104 **b** Resins such as Epon and Spurr harden by polymerization. [Carson & Cappellano, p40]

Answers–Processing

Answers–Processing

The following items (*) have been identified as more appropriate for entry level histotechnologists.

*105 **d** To protect from skin sensitivity, protective gear should be worn when working with chemicals in the electron microscopy lab. [Carson & Cappellano, p40]

*106 **b** Incomplete dehydration of tissues during processing will cause poor staining and lack of nuclear detail after H&E staining. [Carson & Cappellano, p41]

*107 **d** The tissue has been over-dehydrated or over-processed due to long exposure to dehydrants and clearants. [Carson & Cappellano, pp34, 41]

*108 **c** Repeated exposure to epoxy resins may cause dermatitis. [Carson & Cappellano, p40]

*109 **d** Although transparency is not a goal of clearing, it is a result of the clearing steps during processing, due to similar refractive indices. [Bancroft & Gamble, p34]

*110 **d** When the tissue still contains water after clearing steps are complete, the staining results may be uneven staining and poor nuclear detail. [Carson & Cappellano, p41]

*111 **a** Xylene, toluene, and benzene are all hydrocarbons. [Carson & Cappellano, pp34-35]

*112 **c** To maintain tissue morphology of fixed tissue that is to be frozen, the tissue should be infiltrated with 30% sucrose before freezing. [Carson & Cappellano, p51]

*113 **c** Toluene has the lowest viscosity, and will clear tissues most quickly. [Bancroft & Gamble, p84]

*114 **b** Heat increases the penetration and fluid exchange. [Bancroft & Gamble, p84]

*115 **d** Using isopentane chilled to –150°C is the best freezing method for muscle enzyme demonstration. [Carson & Cappellano, pp50, 299]

*116 **c** For demonstration of urate crystals, tissue must be loaded onto the processor in the absolute alcohol step. [Carson & Cappellano, pp7, 244]

*117 **c** Polyethylene glycol (Carbowax) is a water soluble wax which will preserve lipids in tissue. [Carson & Cappellano, p39]

*118 **c** Increasing pressure inside a processing chamber will improve the flow of fluids into tissues. [Bancroft and Gamble, p84; Carson & Cappellano, p67]

*119 **a** Acetone has the lowest viscosity of the choices, making it the most rapid of the dehydration choices. [Bancroft & Gamble, p84]

*120 **c** Isopropanol has the highest viscosity, making it the slowest of the dehydrant choices. [Bancroft & Gamble, p84]

*121 **d** Xylene has the highest viscosity of the clearant choices, making it the slowest. [Bancroft & Gamble, p84]

*122 **b** Washing the decalcified bone marrow specimen in water will stop the action of acid decalcifiers, thus keeping the nuclear basophilia intact. [Carson & Cappellano, p48]

*123 **d** Water-soluble waxes do not require dehydration and clearing. [Carson & Cappellano, p39]

*124 **a** Glycol methacrylate (GMA) will tolerate a small amount of water after processing. [Carson & Cappellano, p40]

*125 **c** Isopropanol is the substitute of choice for ethanol in tissue processing. [Carson & Cappellano, p33]

*126 **c** Double-embedding generally refers to first placing tissue fragments in liquid agar and allowing it to solidify, and then processing the agar-tissue pellet to paraffin wax. [Kiernan, p62]

*127 **c** Glycol methacrylate (GMA) embedding is recommended for very thin sections for light microscopy evaluation. [Carson & Cappellano, p40]

*128 **a** If phosphates from the buffered formalin are not rinsed out before 95% alcohol, the salts will precipitate in the processor. This precipitate may cause difficulties in microtomy. [Carson & Cappellano, p41]

*129 **a** Carbowax is water soluble, and therefore sections cannot be floated on a water bath. [Carson & Cappellano, pp39-40]

*130 **d** Tissue antigens will be denatured by exposure to 70°C paraffin, rendering them unable to be demonstrated. [Bancroft & Gamble, p84]

*131 **c** Because oil red O staining demonstrates lipids in tissue, the tissue cannot be processed to paraffin. Processing to a water soluble wax does not introduce heat or solvents that would dissolve the fats in the sample. [Carson & Cappellano, pp39-40]

*132 **b** Isopropyl alcohol is generally used in microwave processing for both dehydration and clearing, as isopropanol is miscible with paraffin wax. [Carson & Cappellano, p39]

*133 **b** The first step in investigating a temperature that is out of acceptable range is to check the instrument's thermostat to assure that it is set properly. [Carson & Cappellano, pp38, 68, 79]

*134 **c** Oxidative enzyme stains can be done on bone that has been decalcified with a chelation agent such as EDTA. [Carson & Cappellano, p48]

*135 **d** Water soluble wax is the choice to meet the specifications for the research project described. [Carson & Cappellano, pp39-40]

*136 **d** Positively-charged calcium ions are attracted to the negatively-charged cathode. [Carson & Cappellano, p47]

*137 **c** The paraffin bath temperatures are above acceptable range on Wednesday and Thursday, so the tissues processed on those days may show some microtomy artifacts. [Carson & Cappellano, p37]

*138 **a** If bone is not adequately fixed prior to exposure to decalcification acids, the tissue morphology will be adversely affected. [Carson & Cappellano, p46]

*139 **a** Small biopsies, such as gastric, would show the most deleterious effects from the long processing schedule A. [Carson & Cappellano, p37]

*140 **b** The most contaminated (dirty) reagent in each series should be discarded and the subsequent container(s) moved into its place. A fresh (clean) reagent of that series should replace what had been the last container of the series. [Carson & Cappellano, p38]

*141 **c** A fixed needle biopsy would not need further fixation, nor long times in each of the reagents, to achieve adequate processing. [Carson & Cappellano, p38]

*142 **c** When water remains in the tissue into the infiltration step during processing, the staining may be uneven and lack definition. [Carson & Cappellano, pp41, 125]

*143 **a** Agar may be used to hold small fragments of tissue or cellular specimens together during paraffin processing. [Carson & Cappellano, p41]

*144 **a** The recommended method for handling cytologic fluids with spontaneous fibrin clots is to wrap the clot in lens paper and place in a cassette for paraffin processing. [Carson & Cappellano, p324]

*145 **d** The contaminant is pressed so tightly into the tissue specimen that it is obviously a "forceps metastasis," indicating that the forceps were not properly cleaned between specimens. [Carson & Cappellano, pp43-44]

*146 **c** The contaminant is pressed so tightly into the tissue specimen that it is obviously a "forceps metastasis," indicating that the forceps were not properly cleaned between specimens at the embedding table. [Carson & Cappellano, pp43-44]

*147 **b** Eosin will autofluoresce; therefore its presence in tissue will cause autofluorescence interfering with fluorescence techniques such as FISH. [Carson & Cappellano, p32; Kiernan, p117]

*148 **b** Methylene blue is a good colorant for the processor dehydrating solution, especially if sections are to be used for fluorescence techniques such as FISH. [Carson & Cappellano, p32]

Microtomy

The following items have been identified as appropriate for both entry level histotechnicians and histotechnologists.

1 Which of the following is frequently used to soften the exposed face of paraffin embedded tissue that is too hard to section, such as uterine tissue?

   a acid
   b water
   c heat
   d xylene

2 The supplier sent paraffin with a melting point of 50° to 52°C by mistake. When compared to paraffin with a melting point of 55°C, this paraffin will:

   a provide better support for hard tissues
   b yield thinner sections
   c ribbon more easily
   d require a warmer flotation bath

3 A different kind of paraffin is under consideration for use in the laboratory. An important fact to remember is that as the melting point of paraffin is increased, the paraffin:

   a becomes harder
   b provides less support
   c ribbons more easily
   d yields thicker sections

4 To obtain a section of small intestine showing mucosa, submucosa, muscularis externa, and adventitia, the tissue must be embedded:

   a on edge
   b at an angle
   c epithelial surface up
   d mucosal surface down

5 Holes are noted in a frozen section of skeletal muscle. This is most likely the result of

   a too small a clearance angle
   b too cold a cryostat temperature
   c mounting the sections on warm slides
   d freezing the specimen too slowly

6　The angle formed between the block face and the cutting facet of a blade is known as the:

   a rake angle
   b clearance angle
   c bevel angle
   d wedge angle

7　Which of the following will most likely be corrected by soaking a faced block in ice water?

   a lengthwise splits in the sections
   b compressed and jammed sections
   c microscopic chatter
   d mushy sections

8　Which of the following artifacts may be introduced during the flotation process?

   a holes in the tissue
   b the "venetian blind" effect
   c lengthwise splits in the ribbon
   d separation of tissue elements

9　Which of the following embedding procedures involves first infiltrating the tissue with one medium and then embedding it in another?

   a double
   b resin
   c routine
   d vacuum

10　Liver tissue is sectioned in the cryostat and the sections obtained are alternately thick and thin. The most probable cause of this artifact is that the:

   a anti-roll plate is adjusted incorrectly
   b block is too cold
   c blade is dull
   d liver is fatty

11　The type of microtome used for routine paraffin sectioning is a(n):

   a rotary
   b sliding
   c ultramicrotome
   d retracting

12　When cryostat sections are incomplete, or portions of the block do not section, the most likely cause is:

   a sectioning too aggressively
   b incorrect temperature for the tissue
   c incorrect knife angle
   d damaged knife edge

13 The microtomy problem seen below was caused by:

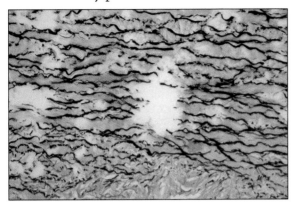

 a a dull blade
 b an incorrect blade angle
 c aggressive sectioning
 d areas of calcification

14 To correct the microtomy problem seen in this section of brain:

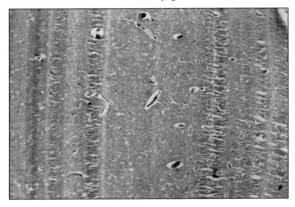

 a change the blade
 b increase the blade tilt
 c clean the blade of paraffin
 d decrease the cutting speed

15 Microorganism contaminants on slides are usually picked up:

 a during ribboning
 b from the staining solution
 c from the flotation bath
 d during slide drying

16 When using an anti-roll plate for frozen sectioning, the plate should be:

 a below the blade edge
 b slightly raised from the blade
 c not parallel to the blade edge
 d fractionally above the blade edge

17   Microscopic examination of an H&E stained section reveals the presence of irregular holes scattered throughout the section. This is most likely caused by:

    a an incorrect blade angle
    b excess section adhesive on the slide
    c the block faced too aggressively
    d the flotation bath not being cleaned between blocks

18   When considering methods for freezing tissue, the coldest and fastest freezing is accomplished by:

    a isopentane cooled by liquid nitrogen
    b dry ice
    c carbon dioxide gas
    d aerosol spray

19   Multiple skin sections should be embedded with the epithelial surfaces facing in:

    a the same direction
    b opposite directions
    c perpendicular directions
    d random directions

20   Microscopic examination of an H&E stained section reveals marked background staining. This is most likely caused by:

    a the use of plus (+) slides
    b excess section adhesive on the slide
    c the flotation bath not being cleaned between blocks
    d section taken immediately after aggressive facing of the block

21   Sections of paraffin embedded tissue show straight lines that appear to be fissures or cuts running at many different angles. This artifact is most likely due to:

    a improper fixation of the tissue
    b introduction of water to the block surface
    c defects in the edge of the blade
    d use of quick-freeze spray to chill the block

22   Hard or bony tissue should be embedded:

    a parallel to the block edge
    b on its edge
    c on its end
    d at an angle

23   Tubular tissue structures should be embedded:

    a flat

    b on edge

    c on end

    d parallel to the block edge

24   To protect the exposed tissue during storage, paraffin blocks may need to be:

    a dipped

    b filed

    c stacked

    d trimmed

25   The microtomy problem see in this image is most likely due to:

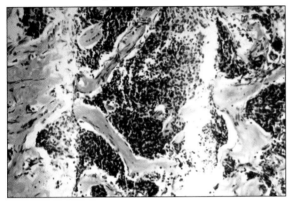

    a the blade not tightly clamped

    b not enough blade tilt

    c a dirty flotation bath

    d aggressive sectioning

26   A microtome is the most likely cause of poor sections when the microtome is:

    a new

    b placed on an incline

    c old or has worn surfaces

    d used by several technicians

27   When compared to routine paraffin microtomy, the tilt of the blade for frozen sectioning is:

    a lesser

    b greater

    c the same

    d insignificant

28   A biopsy of which of the following tissues should be sectioned at 2 micrometers?

    a bladder
    b heart
    c kidney
    d liver

29   Which of the following will cause a split or lengthwise scratch in a paraffin ribbon?

    a debris on the blade edge
    b inadequate processing
    c a blade edge that is too sharp
    d using embedding paraffin with the wrong melting point

30   The purpose of embedding tissue in paraffin is to:

    a preserve its antigenicity
    b stabilize proteins
    c provide support
    d remove water from the cells

31   Which of the following groups of special stains requires sections cut at 8 - 10 μm?

    a Congo red, Lieb crystal violet, Bielschowsky
    b Kinyoun, Snook, oil red O
    c von Kossa, Fontana-Masson, Sudan black B
    d Verhoeff-van Gieson, aldehyde fuchsin, Masson trichrome

32   During sectioning of a block of uterine tissue, alternate thick and thin zones are observed. This is most likely caused by:

    a improper embedding
    b inadequate processing
    c vibration of the blade
    d non-parallel block edges

33   Microscopic examination of an H&E stained section reveals the presence of extraneous epithelial cells. This is most likely caused by:

    a squamous cells from dry skin of hands
    b excess section adhesive on the slide
    c sections being taken immediately after "rough facing" of the block
    d the flotation bath not being cleaned between blocks

34   Disposable blades should be discarded:

    a by incineration
    b by wrapping with tape and placing in wastepaper basket
    c in a separate "sharps" container
    d via the garbage disposal

35   Crooked ribbons result when the:

    a horizontal edges of the block are not parallel
    b block is aggressively sectioned
    c the clearance angle is incorrect
    d room temperature is too warm

36   For which of the following stains should sections be cut at 10-15 μm?

    a Jones (PAMS)
    b thioflavin T
    c periodic acid-Schiff
    d Luxol fast blue

37   Most ovens used for drying slides are commonly maintained at a temperature:

    a 40°C
    b 50°C
    c 60°C
    d 70°C

38   Which of the following blade profiles is recommended for frozen sectioning?

    a biconcave
    b planoconcave
    c low
    d high

39   One cause of the artifact seen below is:

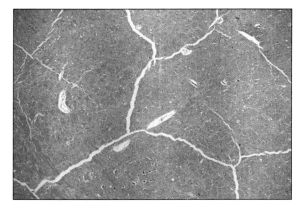

    a a defect in the blade edge
    b drying at too high a temperature
    c worn microtome part
    d using a fluorocarbon spray on the block

40   The orientation of a specimen for embedding should be decided during:

    a fixation
    b grossing
    c processing
    d surgical removal

41   When cutting 30 μm sections of fixed brain tissue in a –20°C cryostat, the
      sections fragment at the blade edge. This problem could most likely be prevented
      by:

      a lowering the cryostat temperature to –30°C
      b raising the cryostat temperature to –7°C
      c freezing the tissue in liquid nitrogen
      d using the anti-roll plate

42   Unfixed cryostat sections are most commonly attached to slides by:

      a placing them in water and then floating onto clean slides
      b brushing them onto a clean, very cold slide
      c picking them up from the blade onto an albuminized slide
      d picking them up from the blade onto a clean, warm slide

43   When paraffin with a 54° to 56°C melting point is used for embedding, the
      temperature of the flotation bath should fall within which of the following
      temperature (°C) ranges?

      a 41 to 45
      b 46 to 50
      c 51 to 55
      d 56 to 60

44   Routine cryostat sections are usually cut at:

      a –10°C
      b –20°C
      c –30°C
      d –40°C

45   Paraffin sections are being lifted from the blade on the upstroke. This is probably
      because the:

      a blade is too sharp
      b blade tilt is incorrect
      c paraffin is too cold
      d specimen is too hard

46   One of the causes of the microtomy problem seen in this image is:

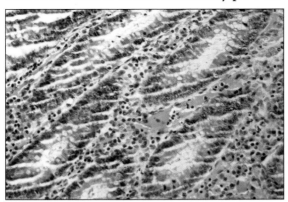

     a aggressive facing of the block
     b the blade is too sharp
     c defects in the blade edge
     d an excessively dehydrated block

47   Cryostat sections of fixed tissue are tending to float off the slides during staining. This problem can be prevented by:

     a coating the slides with an adhesive mixture
     b heating the slides over a Bunsen burner
     c picking up the sections on a room temperature slide
     d sectioning at a warmer temperature

48   For ONLY 1 layer of nuclei to be seen in a section, the section should be no thicker than:

     a 3 μm
     b 5 μm
     c 7 μm
     d 9 μm

49   The College of American Pathologists (CAP) recommends that a cryostat in daily use be decontaminated:

     a daily
     b weekly
     c biweekly
     d monthly

50   To prevent the formation of a thick layer of paraffin on the bottom of the mold during embedding, the tissue must be:

     a embedded quickly and precisely
     b handled carefully and slowly
     c heated directly on a hot plate
     d reoriented several times

51   The tissue surface to be cut should be placed against which aspect of the embedding mold?

   a bottom
   b edge
   c side
   d top

52   Paraffin is converted from the fluid state to the solid state by:

   a crystallization
   b evaporation
   c polymerization
   d sublimation

53   Routine paraffin sections are cut at what micrometer (micron, μm) setting?

   a 1 to 2
   b 4 to 5
   c 7 to 8
   d 10 to 12

54   As the block face is trimmed, the blade digs into the tissue and gouges out a chunk. The most probable cause of this problem is that the:

   a block is too cool
   b blade is dull
   c block is loose in the chuck
   d cutting stroke is too rapid

55   Nuclear bubbling is seen on an H&E section. This most likely was caused by:

   a overfixing the tissue
   b drying undrained slides at too high a temperature
   c cutting sections at the wrong micrometer setting
   d adding adhesive to the flotation bath

56   The clearance angle used with most microtome blades for paraffin sectioning is:

   a 3 to 8 degrees
   b 15 to 23 degrees
   c 27 to 32 degrees
   d 42 to 45 degrees

57   Microscopic examination of an H&E stained section reveals the presence of extraneous tumor cells. This is most likely caused by:

   a squamous cells shed by hands put in the flotation bath
   b excess section adhesive on the slide
   c sections taken immediately after aggressive facing of the block
   d the flotation bath not being cleaned between blocks

58   Layered structures such as cyst wall and gallbladder should be embedded:

     a lengthwise
     b on edge
     c on end
     d parallel to block side

59   During paraffin embedding, it is noted that several sections appear soft and mushy. This is most likely due to:

     a inadequate processing
     b prolonged fixation
     c paraffin that is too warm
     d the type of tissue processed

60   Which of the following is necessary to ensure a straight ribbon?

     a horizontal sides of the block must be parallel.
     b vertical sides of the block must be parallel.
     c horizontal and vertical sides of the block must be parallel.
     d the microtome wheel must be rotated rapidly.

61   Microscopic examination of stained slides shows bacilli on, but not in, the tissue sections. The most probable cause of this contaminant is that:

     a excess albumin on the slides attracted microorganisms
     b excess gelatin was added to the water bath
     c the flotation bath was not cleaned from the previous day
     d there is excess poly-L-lysine on the slides

62   Paraffin used for embedding should be how many degrees centigrade above the melting point of the medium?

     a 0 to 1
     b 2 to 4
     c 5 to 7
     d 8 to 10

63   Sections of brain that tend to wash off slides during staining can be adhered to slides by coating the section/slide with:

     a Carbowax
     b polyethylene glycol
     c paraffin
     d poly-L-lysine

64   Frozen sections are required when:

     a excellent morphologic detail is required
     b immediate microscopic evaluation is required
     c demonstration of cytoplasmic IgG is to be done
     d retinal pathology is suspected

65 When frozen sections bunch up at the knife edge and cannot be flattened, one explanation is that:

    a the blade is too warm
    b the chuck is not clamped firmly
    c tissue is not parallel to the blade edge
    d the microtome is not advancing properly

66 One cause of sections sticking to each other or to parts of the microtome is:

    a air currents
    b a radio operating in the room
    c static electricity
    d the wrong air temperature

67 Part of the preventive maintenance for the cryostat should include:

    a keeping the refrigerant coils free of dust
    b oiling of the microtome daily
    c decontamination of the cryostat daily
    d pick up tissue shavings every other day

68 The microtomy artifact seen in the center of this image is the result of:

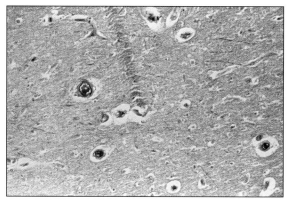

    a a dull blade
    b too large a clearance angle
    c a defect in the blade edge
    d a small focus of calcium

69 Which of the following problems will be seen in paraffin sections that are floated out on a flotation bath that is too cold?

    a cracks
    b folds
    c separations
    d stretching

70   During microtomy, several successive paraffin sections are compressed and wrinkled. The most appropriate action is to:

    a change to a new blade
    b increase the rapidity of cutting
    c check the paraffin melting point
    d increase the flotation bath temperature

71   Refer to the following data:

cryostat temperature chart	
day	**temperature (°C)**
Monday	−20
Tuesday	−15
Wednesday	−18
Thursday	−23
Friday	−26

    On which day would sectioning of breast tissue be most difficult?

    a Monday
    b Tuesday
    c Thursday
    d Friday

72   Which of the following could be substituted for gelatin as an additive to the flotation bath?

    a aminoalkylsilane
    b chromium potassium sulfate
    c poly-L-lysine
    d agar

73   During microtomy, it is noted that a faced block has a central area that is soft and mushy. This tissue should have been:

    a chilled longer before facing
    b cut thicker at the grossing table
    c left in paraffin longer
    d reprocessed before embedding

74   Lymph node tissue shatters when sectioned in a cryostat maintained at −20°C. The most appropriate action is to:

    a switch to an unused part of the blade
    b increase the blade tilt
    c chill the block with a spray coolant
    d warm the block slightly

75   For good demonstration of myelin sheaths, paraffin sections should be:

   a floated on a cool water bath
   b cut 10 to 15 μm thick
   c coated with celloidin
   d dried at room temperature

76   In paraffin microtomy, knowledge of the tissue type and possible disease process present in the tissue may be important because it may change the requirements in:

   a clearance angle
   b section thickness
   c flotation medium
   d blade temperature

77   Prominent peripheral chatter is obtained on sections of a paraffin block that has been routinely fixed and processed. This can probably be corrected by recutting the block:

   a after soaking it in ice water
   b using a faster cutting speed
   c after re-embedding in a different paraffin
   d using a greater clearance angle

78   Slides used for mounting cryostat frozen sections should be kept at the same temperature as the:

   a tissue
   b blade
   c operator
   d room

79   Paraffin sections should be cut at 2 micrometers when studying:

   a basement membranes
   b myelin
   c amyloid
   d nerve fibers

80   The tissue block fails to advance during the preparation of frozen sections. This probably could be corrected by:

   a changing the blade angle
   b replacing the blade
   c decreasing the chamber temperature
   d cleaning and oiling the microtome

81   An H&E stained lymph node section reveals overlapping nuclei. This indicates that the section is most likely:

    a   overstained with hematoxylin
    b   too thick
    c   of an abnormal node
    d   appropriately sectioned

82   The material of choice for immunofluorescence microscopy and enzyme histochemical studies is:

    a   paraffin sections
    b   cryostat sections
    c   air-dried imprints
    d   alcohol-fixed imprints

83   When a femoral head is sectioned, the marrow portion sections satisfactorily but the cortex fragments. The most probable cause of this problem is that the:

    a   decalcifying agent was too strong
    b   embedding medium is too hard
    c   decalcifying agent was not washed out
    d   compact bone is underdecalcified

84   A fingernail has been fixed in formalin, routinely processed, and embedded in paraffin. The tissue is very hard and sections are difficult to obtain. Sectioning quality will be improved and tissue components will be BEST preserved and demonstrated by gently facing the block and:

    a   soaking in water
    b   warming the block slightly
    c   soaking in a solution that softens keratin
    d   treating with a decalcifying fluid

85   Nuclear bubbling artifact may be caused by:

    a   leaving section too long on the flotation bath
    b   using too much adhesive in the flotation bath
    c   placing the slide in a hot dryer without allowing to drain
    d   sectioning too rapidly

86   According to the Histology Quality Improvement Program, the most common microtomy artifact is:

    a   wavy sections
    b   holes in the section
    c   air bubbles
    d   winkles and folds

87 Of the following, the most common cause of tears and/or section fragmentation is:

   a incomplete fixation and processing
   b flotation bath too cold
   c dull microtome blade
   d worn microtome parts

88 The use of coolant sprays during sectioning may result in:

   a wavy sections
   b fragmented sections
   c parched earth appearance
   d chatter or microvibration

89 A very serious microtomy artifact in the histopathology laboratory is:

   a squamous debris on section
   b contaminant from another tissue source
   c folds or wrinkles
   d compressed sections

90 The artifact seen in the image below most likely could have been corrected by:

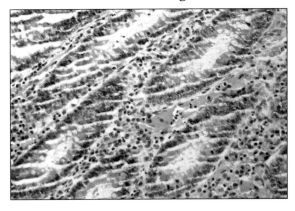

   a increasing the blade tilt
   b sectioning more rapidly
   c soaking the faced block with moist cotton
   d cutting deeper in the block

The following items (*) have been identified as more appropriate for entry level histotechnologists.

*91 The preferred knife for cutting thin sections of epoxy embedded tissue is:

   a glass
   b steel
   c diamond
   d ceramic

*92 If chatter is noted in several microscopic sections, all of the following should be checked EXCEPT:

   a overdehydrated tissue
   b a dull microtome blade
   c an overextended block holder shaft
   d too little blade tilt

*93 A section of skeletal muscle has been frozen in isopentane and liquid nitrogen, but numerous holes are seen in the H&E stained sections. This problem is most commonly caused by:

   a non-isometrically fixed muscle tissue
   b sectioning too soon after freezing
   c leaving in the isopentane too long
   d isopentane that is not cold enough

*94 "Thick" sections for electron microscopy, or sections to be viewed with the light microscope, are cut at:

   a 4 to 6 nanometers
   b 60 to 70 nanometers
   c 0.5 to 1.0 micrometers
   d 4 to 6 micrometers

*95 For diagnostic purposes, the type of biopsy tissue seen below should be cut at:

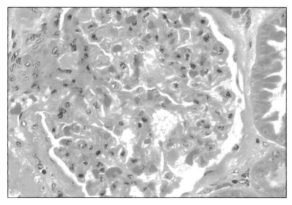

   a 2 μm
   b 4 μm
   c 6 μm
   d 8 μm

*96 When cutting frozen sections, the tissue is frequently becoming detached from the chuck. The MOST likely cause is that:

   a gum tragacanth was used as the embedding medium
   b the chuck was at room temperature when embedding medium applied
   c the chuck was too cold when embedding medium applied
   d the embedding medium was at room temperature

*97   Sectioning fixed tissue with a cryostat may be improved by:

    a chilling in the refrigerator before freezing
    b freezing the tissue very slowly
    c using gum tragacanth to mount the tissue on the object disc
    d infiltrating with 30% sucrose before freezing

*98   One technician consistently produces sections that show the following artifact. The problem is most likely caused by:

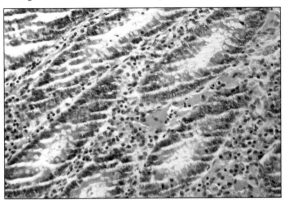

    a cutting too rapidly
    b incomplete dehydration
    c too little blade tilt
    d flotation bath too hot

*99   A section of skeletal muscle has been frozen in isopentane and liquid nitrogen, but numerous holes are seen in the H&E stained sections. This problem might be prevented in the future by:

    a freezing in liquid nitrogen alone
    b sectioning immediately after freezing
    c making sure that the isopentane is at –150°C
    d isometrically fixing the section of muscle

*100 The supervisor notices that one microtomist consistently is sectioning by rocking the hand wheel on the microtome. The supervisor should:

    a take no action; this is an acceptable practice
    b suggest to the microtomist that this practice may lead to thicker sections
    c suggest to the microtomist that the chair height be adjusted
    d counsel the microtomist that this practice may lead to carpal tunnel syndrome

*101 The pathologist requests a naphthol AS-D chloroacetate esterase stain. Of the following, the most appropriate section for this stain is:

    a unfixed frozen
    b formalin fixed frozen
    c formalin fixed paraffin
    d formic acid decalcified bone marrow

*102 The SOP for the following stain should indicate that the sections are to be cut at:

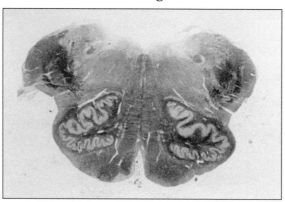

    a 2 - 4 μm
    b 5 - 8 μm
    c 10 - 15 μm
    d 16 - 20 μm

*103 During the sectioning of plastic blocks with an ultramicrotome, scratches are seen in the sections. The problem is most likely caused by:

    a paraffin embedded and sectioned at 4 - 5 μm
    b paraffin embedded and sectioned at 10 - 15 μm
    c unfixed, frozen and sectioned at 4 - 5 μm
    d unfixed, frozen and sectioned at 8 - 10 μm

*104 The microtome used for electron microscopy is called a(n):

    a rotary microtome
    b sliding microtome
    c freezing microtome
    d ultramicrotome

*105 For staining, muscle biopsies submitted for diagnosis should be:

    a paraffin embedded and sectioned at 4 - 5 μm
    b paraffin embedded and sectioned at 10 - 15 μm
    c unfixed, frozen, and sectioned at 2 - 5 μm
    d unfixed, frozen, and sectioned at 8 - 10 μm

*106 The square object seen on the far left of this cassette label is a:

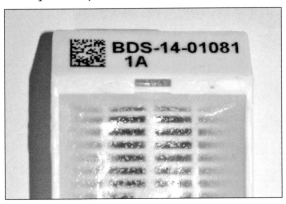

   a hospital logo
   b linear bar code
   c 2D bar code
   d 3D bar code

*107 One histotechnician routinely produces sections that contain the artifact seen below. What is the most appropriate question for the technician?

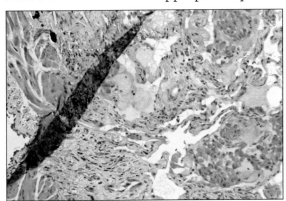

   a is the knife tilt correct?
   b how often is the blade changed?
   c how fast is the cutting speed?
   d are the ribbons being stretched?

*108 Glass knives are being made for cutting thin resin-embedded sections. They should be broken:

   a as needed
   b weekly
   c bimonthly
   d monthly

*109 During the sectioning of plastic blocks with an ultramicrotome, alternating thick and thin sections are obtained. The problem is most likely caused by:

    a dirt
    b a wet block face
    c a loose blade
    d an incorrect water level

*110 A research project requires that extra large sections be cut. The BEST microtome for this purpose is of what type:

    a rotary
    b sliding
    c rocking
    d vibrating

*111 Coating a slide with a basic polymer in which a chemical reaction occurs leaving the amino groups linked by covalent bonds to the silicon atoms of the glass is descriptive of:

    a poly-L-lysine slide coating
    b plus slide creation
    c aminoalkysilane-treated slides
    d a cytologic technique

*112 Glass knives are used for sectioning tissue embedded in:

    a celloidin
    b glycol methacrylate only
    c epoxy resin only
    d glycol methacrylate and epoxy resin

*113 Sections for the stain shown in the image below will show yellow birefringence instead of apple green if the sections are cut at:

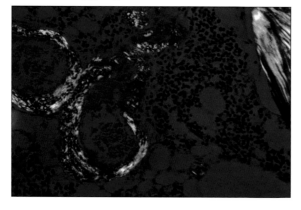

    a 2 microns
    b 5 microns
    c 8 microns
    d 15 microns

*114 When considering the purchase of a new tissue processor, all of the following should be considered EXCEPT:

    a the rigidity of protocols
    b reagent usage
    c necessity of validation
    d space and ventilation requirements

*115 Undecalcified bone can be sectioned most easily when embedded in:

    a celloidin
    b plastic
    c water soluble wax
    d paraffin

*116 Before using new equipment, all of the following must be verified EXCEPT:

    a side-by- side comparisons
    b availability of proper electrical wattage
    c need for dedicated ventilation or plumbing
    d need for LIS or internet connectivity

*117 A technician is having trouble getting all paraffin embedded blocks to ribbon. Examination reveals that the tissues were embedded in 62°C melting-point paraffin and the room temperature is 25°C. Which of the following actions should correct the problem in the future?

    a immediately ordering some lower melting point paraffin
    b soaking faced blocks in ice water before ribboning
    c warming faced blocks before ribboning
    d lowering the room temperature

*118 The instrumentation QC manual states that flotation baths must be emptied and thoroughly cleaned on Fridays. The bath may be refilled and additional adhesive may be added as needed during the week. This procedure:

    a may be considered as satisfactory
    b should be changed to read "emptied and cleaned twice a week"
    c may lead to bacterial contamination of microscopic sections
    d will probably increase section loss during staining

*119 Periodic acid methenamine silver (PAMS) stained kidney sections reveal well impregnated basement membranes. However, within the individual glomeruli the membranes overlap and cannot be evaluated as separate structures. This could be corrected by cutting sections at:

    a 2 to 3 micrometers
    b 5 to 6 micrometers
    c 8 to 9 micrometers
    d 13 to 15 micrometers

*120 A microscopic section of liver tissue shows numerous irregular holes throughout the tissue. This is most likely because:

    a the holes are portal triads
    b liver is difficult to cut
    c fixation has been prolonged
    d sectioning technique was poor

*121 The knife required for sectioning glycol methacrylate tissue is made of:

    a aluminum
    b steel
    c glass
    d diamond

*122 Successive cryostat sections catch on one area in the middle of the anti-roll plate. The most likely cause is that the anti-roll plate is:

    a warmer than the blade
    b colder than the blade
    c improperly adjusted
    d damaged

*123 Amyloid control sections stained with crystal violet fail to show the typical metachromasia of the amyloid. One possible explanation is that the:

    a sections were freshly cut
    b sections were cut at 4 μm
    c an aqueous mountant was used
    d the staining solution was acidified

*124 A ribbon of paraffin embedded brain tissue is floated on the water bath. Small holes are noted in the first section and decrease in size in subsequent sections. The most appropriate action is to:

    a melt the block and re-embed the tissue
    b resharpen the blade
    c decrease the water bath temperature
    d cut and discard ribbons until the holes disappear

*125 When comparing the cut sections to the block, the image seen below expresses a problem. The supervisor should check all of the following EXCEPT:

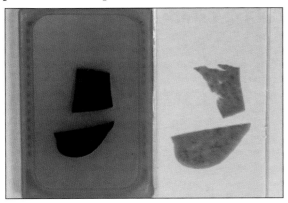

  a embedding techniques
  b are microtomy sections taken too early
  c consistent microtome blade defects
  d are sections taken after tissue is cut away

*126 Microscopic evaluation of a stained section has the following appearance. The section:

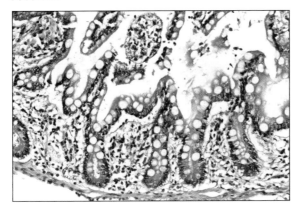

  a has been cut with a dull knife
  b shows cell shrinkage
  c demonstrates a compression problem
  d does not show any problem

*127 The problem seen in the image below most likely could have been prevented by:

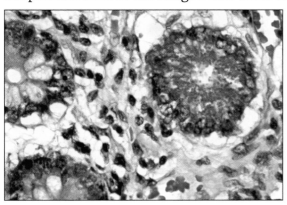

    a allowing the slide to drain longer before drying
    b sectioning with a sharper blade
    c floating on a warmer flotation bath
    d retracting the block holder shaft

*128 The pathologists are complaining that the Congo red stained sections are showing faint red instead of apple green birefringence. The most likely cause is that the microtomists are:

    a drying the sections at too high a temperature
    b floating the sections too long on the flotation bath
    c cutting the sections at the routine 4-5 micrometers
    d not chilling the block sufficiently

*129 The problem seen in the cryostat image below can be corrected by:

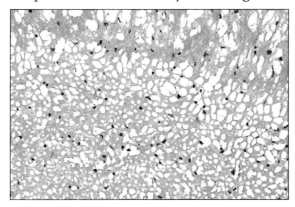

    a instituting a different method of freezing tissue
    b adjusting the anti-roll plate
    c ensuring the use of a high profile blade
    d decreasing the blade tilt

*130 Nuclear bubbling may be caused by all of the following EXCEPT:

   a incomplete fixation before processing
   b microwave drying of slides
   c overnight drying of slides
   d insufficient draining of slides before drying

*131 The microtomist responsible for cutting the section seen below should be counseled for:

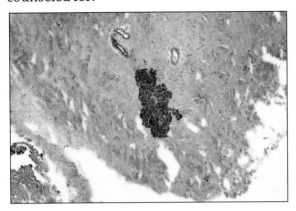

   a cutting sections too thick
   b not cleaning the flotation bath between blocks
   c using a blade with a defective edge
   d insufficient draining of slides before drying

*132 The pathologist notes numerous air bubbles trapped under the sections. The supervisor, when notified about the problem should caution the microtomist to:

   a float sections for a longer period of time
   b dry slides at a lower temperature
   c allow the flotation bath water to stand overnight
   d drain slides well before drying

*133 One microtomist often produces slides with the following problem. This is because the microtomist is:

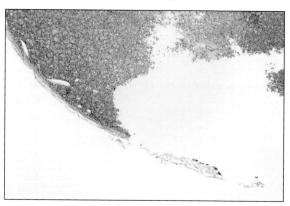

   a picking up sections too early
   b not cleaning the flotation bath properly
   c drying slides at too hot a temperature
   d using a blade with a defective edge

*134 The pathologist is complaining about the number of floater contaminants on the H&E-stained sections. The most likely source of the contamination is the:

   a flotation bath
   b automated "dip and dunk" stainer
   c embedding procedures
   d grossing table

The following items have been identified as appropriate for both entry level histotechnicians and histotechnologists.

1	b	17	c	33	a	49	b	65	a	81	b
2	c	18	a	34	c	50	a	66	c	82	b
3	a	19	a	35	a	51	a	67	a	83	d
4	a	20	b	36	d	52	a	68	d	84	c
5	d	21	d	37	c	53	b	69	b	85	c
6	b	22	d	38	d	54	c	70	a	86	d
7	c	23	c	39	d	55	b	71	b	87	a
8	d	24	a	40	b	56	a	72	d	88	c
9	a	25	a	41	b	57	d	73	d	89	b
10	c	26	c	42	d	58	b	74	d	90	c
11	a	27	b	43	b	59	a	75	b		
12	b	28	c	44	b	60	a	76	b		
13	c	29	a	45	b	61	c	77	a		
14	a	30	c	46	d	62	b	78	d		
15	c	31	a	47	a	63	d	79	a		
16	d	32	c	48	b	64	b	80	d		

The following items (*) have been identified as more appropriate for entry level histotechnologists.

*91	c	*99	c	*107	d	*115	b	*123	b	*131	b
*92	d	*100	d	*108	a	*116	a	*124	d	*132	c
*93	d	*101	c	*109	c	*117	a	*125	c	*133	a
*94	c	*102	c	*110	b	*118	c	*126	b	*134	b
*95	a	*103	a	*111	b	*119	a	*127	a		
*96	c	*104	d	*112	d	*120	d	*128	c		
*97	d	*105	d	*113	d	*121	c	*129	a		
*98	a	*106	c	*114	c	*122	d	*130	c		

 ISBN 978-089189-6494   ©ASCP 2016

The following items have been identified as appropriate for both entry level histotechnicians and histotechnologists.

1   **b**   Prolonged soaking of a faced block in water, or exposing the block surface to running tap water for 30 minutes will often allow obtaining ribbons from tissue that is hard to section. [Bancroft & Gamble, p96]

2   **c**   The lower the melting point of the paraffin, the easier it is to obtain ribbons. [Carson & Cappellano, p42]

3   **a**   The higher the melting point of the paraffin, the harder it becomes. Higher melting point paraffins provide better support for hard tissue. [Carson & Cappellano, p42]

4   **a**   The mucosa, submucosa, muscularis externa, and adventitia are the layers of the small intestinal wall that should be seen if the section is embedded on edge. [Carson & Cappellano, pp42-43]

5   **d**   If tissue is frozen too slowly, the water in the tissue will freeze and form ice crystals of a size proportional to the speed of freezing. When thawed, the ice crystals melt and produce the freeze artifact known as holes. [Carson & Cappellano, pp50-51]

6   **b**   The angle formed between the block face and the cutting facet of a blade is known as the clearance angle. That angle and the condition of the blade edge are the most important factors in obtaining good sections. [Carson & Cappellano, p59]

7   **c**   Microscopic chatter often results from overdehydrated tissue; soaking the faced block in ice water will help restore moisture to the tissue and make obtaining an artifact free section easier. [Carson & Cappellano, p64]

8   **d**   Allowing tissue to remain too long on the flotation bath may cause over expansion of the section and the separation of tissue elements. [Brown, p24]

9   **a**   Double embedding refers to first infiltrating the tissue with one medium (such as gelatin) and the embedding it in another (such as paraffin). [Carson & Cappellano, p41; Kiernan, p62]

10   **c**   A dull blade will cause alternate thick and thin frozen sections. [Brown, p20]

11   **a**   The rotary microtome is used for routine paraffin sectioning; the sliding for large blocks and celloidin embedded tissues; the ultramicrotome and retracting microtome for electron microscopy. [Bancroft & Gamble, p93; Carson & Cappellano, p58]

12   **b**   When cryostat sections are incomplete, the most likely cause is that the cryostat is not at the correct temperature for the tissue being sectioned. Some tissue components like fat or other lipid rich tissues will require a much colder temperature in order to section properly. [Brown, p34]

13   **c**   The holes in the section were caused by facing the block too aggressively. [Carson & Cappellano, p61]

14   **a**   The many knife lines seen in this section were caused by defects in the blade edge; the blade should be changed. [Brown, p18]

15   **c**   If the flotation bath is not scrupulously cleaned at the end of each day, microorganisms may grow in the bath. Also organisms have been reported in tap water, gelatin, and Elmer's glue used in the bath. One should always be aware of the possibility of flotation bath contamination. [Carson & Cappellano, p72]

16   **d**   The anti-roll plate should extend fractionally above the knife edge. [Carson & Cappellano, p67]

17   **c**   Aggressive facing of the block will cause small spicules of tissue to be pulled from the block face leaving holes in the tissue sections. [Carson & Cappellano, p60]

18   **a**   The coldest and fastest freezing is accomplished by isopentane cooled by liquid nitrogen. Only liquid nitrogen can achieve colder temperatures, but it will impede freezing by the formation of gas bubbles around tissue suspended directly in it. [Bancroft & Gamble, p50]

19   **a**   Multiple skin sections should be embedded so that all epithelial surfaces face in the same direction. [Carson & Cappellano, p43]

20   **b**   If too much adhesive is applied directly to the slide, it may stain. [Carson & Cappellano, p73]

21   **d**   Aerosol sprays used on the block face during microtomy may cause fractures in the block face; this will be seen as fissures running in multiple directions in the sections. [Carson & Cappellano, p71]

22   **d**   Hard or bony tissue will section more easily if it is embedded at an angle. [Carson & Cappellano, p43]

23   **c**   Tubular tissues should be embedded on end. [Carson & Cappellano, p43]

24   **a**   Blocks may need to be dipped, or resealed, to protect the tissue from moisture, air drying, or insects. [Bancroft & Gamble, p479]

25   **a**   The washboarding, or thick and thin areas within a single section, may be due to a blade that is not tightly clamped. It also can be cause by too much knife tilt, worn or loose microtome parts, a dull knife, and very dense or compact tissue. [Carson & Cappellano, p62]

26   **c**   A microtome is most likely the cause of poor sections when the microtome is old or has worn surfaces. [Bancroft & Gamble, p15; Carson & Cappellano, p62]

27   **b**   The blade tilt for cutting frozen sections is very significant and is greater than that used for paraffin sectioning. [Carson & Cappellano, p66]

28   **c**   Kidney biopsies are usually sectioned at 2 μm. [Carson & Cappellano, p59]

29   **a**   Debris or paraffin on the blade edge can cause lengthwise splits or scratches in paraffin ribbons. [Brown, p18]

30   **c**   Embedding in paraffin provides support for tissue, so that thin sections may be cut. [Carson & Cappellano, p37]

31   **a**   Stains for amyloid (Lieb crystal violet, Congo red) and for several neural stains (Bielschowsky) require sections cut at 8 - 10 μm. [Carson & Cappellano, pp154-156, 196]

32   **c**   One cause of thick and thin zones in tissue sections is vibration of the blade; this most commonly occurs in very hard tissue. This may also result from loose or worn microtome parts and either the blade or block not being tightly clamped. [Carson & Cappellano, p64]

33   **a**   Extraneous epithelial cells may occur in the flotation bath from dandruff or shedding of cells from very dry skin as the fingers touch the bath. [Brown, pp21-22]

34   **c**   Disposable blades should be discarded in separate "sharps" container. [Carson & Cappellano, p59]

35   **a**   If the horizontal (top and bottom) edges of the block are not parallel, a crooked ribbon will result. [Carson & Cappellano, p60]

36   **d**   Sections should be cut at 10-15 μm for the best demonstration of the myelin sheath (Luxol fast blue and Weil stains). [Carson & Cappellano, pp204-206]

37   **c**   Ovens used for drying paraffin sections commonly are maintained at 60°C, which is just above the melting point of the paraffin. [Carson & Cappellano, p71]

38   **d**   High profile blades are recommended for frozen sectioning. [Carson & Cappellano, p66]

39   **d**   One cause of the parched earth artifact seen in the image is the use of fluorocarbon spray on the face of the block; this artifact can also be caused when improperly processed tissue is floated on the flotation bath or if the flotation bath is too hot. [Carson & Cappellano, p71]

40   **b**   The orientation of tissue sections should be decided at the time of grossing. When necessary, there are several ways of indicating the surface to be placed up in the block. [Carson & Cappellano, p42]

41   **b**   Brain tissue cuts most easily at −7° to −10°C, so the temperature of the cryostat should be raised. [Bancroft & Gamble, p101]

42   **d**   Cryostat sections are picked up on a clean warm slide. [Bancroft & Gamble, p100]

43   **b**   The temperature of the flotation bath should be 46°C to 50°C, as the bath is usually maintained 5°C to 10°C below the melting point of the paraffin. [Carson & Cappellano, p71]

44   **b**   Routine cryostat sections are usually cut at −20°C. [Carson & Cappellano, p66]

45   **b**   Sections will lift from the blade as the block is raised if the tilt of the knife is incorrect, usually too little tilt. [Carson & Cappellano, p62]

46 **d** Chatter, or microscopic vibration, is most commonly caused by overdehydration of the tissue during processing. It can also be caused by cutting too rapidly. [Carson & Cappellano, p64]

47 **a** Frozen sections of fixed tissue will not adhere well to clean slides, so a slide coated with an adhesive mixture, or charged slides should be used. [Bancroft & Gamble, p101]

48 **b** Sections any thicker than 4-5 μm will show more than one layer of nuclei; these sections are too thick for routine H&E staining. [Carson & Cappellano, p59]

49 **b** The CAP recommends that a cryostat in daily use be decontaminated once a week. [Carson & Cappellano, p67]

50 **a** Tissue should be embedded quickly and precisely, keeping the paraffin melted until all pieces are in the mold and then pressing down lightly on the tissue and chilling until adherence to the bottom of the mold is achieved. [Brown, p11]

51 **a** The tissue surface to be cut should be placed against the bottom of the embedding mold. [Carson & Cappellano, p42]

52 **a** Paraffin crystallizes as it is cooled, and quick cooling of the embedded tissue block ensure a small crystalline structure, thus producing fewer artifacts during microtomy. [Carson & Cappellano, p44]

53 **b** Most routine paraffin sections are cut at a microtomy setting of 3-5 μm. [Carson & Cappellano, p59]

54 **c** When the microtome blade bites into the tissue during sectioning, the most likely cause is that either the block or the blade is not clamped securely. [Carson & Cappellano, p63]

55 **b** If undrained slides are dried at too high a temperature, nuclear bubbling is likely the result. [Carson & Cappellano, p76]

56 **a** The clearance angle used with most microtome blades for paraffin sectioning is 3° - 8°. [Carson & Cappellano, p59]

57 **d** Extraneous tumor cells were picked up from a previous case, because the flotation bath was not "skimmed" or cleaned between blocks or cases. [Carson & Cappellano, p74]

58 **b** Layered structures such a cyst wall or gallbladder should be embedded on edge. [Carson & Cappellano, p42]

59 **a** Soft and mushy tissues noted during paraffin embedding are most likely the result of inadequate processing. [Carson & Cappellano, p45]

60 **a** The horizontal sides of the block must be parallel to ensure a straight ribbon. [Carson & Cappellano, p60]

61 **c** The flotation bath should be carefully and thoroughly dried at the end of each day, and allowed to dry overnight; a dirty bath may encourage the growth of organism if left overnight. [Carson & Cappellano, p73]

62 **b** Paraffin for embedding should be maintained 2°C -4°C above the melting point of the paraffin. [Carson & Cappellano, p79]

63 **d** Poly-L-lysine coated slides are used for mounting tissues that tend to wash off during staining, and also for frozen sections of fixed tissues. [Carson & Cappellano, p73]

64 **b** Frozen sections are required for immediate microscopic evaluation. [Bancroft & Gamble, p102; Carson & Cappellano, p50]

65 **a** A warm knife will cause a frozen section to bunch up and not slide under an anti-roll plate, or be flattened with a brush. [Brown, p32]

66 **c** Static electricity will cause paraffin sections to fly and stick to each other or to parts of the microtome. [Carson & Cappellano, p66]

67 **a** Preventive maintenance for the cryostat should include keeping the refrigerant coils free of dust. [Carson & Cappellano, p67]

68 **d** The microtomy artifact seen the center appears to be a knife line, but because it does not go completely through the section, but begins in the middle, it is caused by a small focus of calcium. A knife line, or one caused by a defect in the blade edge would go completely across the section, as the fine line seen on the left does. [Carson & Cappellano, p60]

69 **b** Tissue will not float out properly if the flotation bath is too cold, and wrinkles and folds will be the result. [Brown, p17]

70 **a** One of the causes of compressed, or wrinkled, sections is a dull knife. The blade should be changed. [Carson & Cappellano, p64]

71 **b** Breast tissue, especially if it contains any fat, will not section well at the warmer cryostat temperature, such as that seen on Tuesday. The cryostat should be at least –20°C to –25°C. [Bancroft & Gamble, p101]

72 **d** Agar may be added to the flotation bath instead of gelatin. [Carson & Cappellano, p72]

73 **d** The block has been inadequately processed and it should be reprocessed. This should have been caught at the embedding table, and the tissue reprocessed at that point. [Carson & Cappellano, p45]

74 **d** Warming the block should allow better sectioning. When shattering occurs, it usually indicates that the block is too cold. [Bancroft & Gamble, p100; Brown, p30]

75 **b** Sections for the demonstration of myelin sheaths should be cut at 10 - 15 μm. [Carson & Cappellano, pp204-206]

76 **b** Knowledge of the tissue type or the disease process is important because it may change the requirements in section thickness. [Carson & Cappellano, p59]

77 **a** Peripheral chatter is usually the result of overdehydration; soaking the faced block in ice water should aid in obtaining better sections. [Carson & Cappellano, p64]

78 **d** Room temperature slides should be used for picking up cryostat sections. [Bancroft & Gamble, p100]

79 **a** Slides should be cut at 2 μm when studying basement membranes. [Carson & Cappellano, p180]

Answers–Microtomy

80 **d** In older model cryostats, ice formation is not uncommon within the advance mechanism of the microtome; this can only be corrected by defrosting, cleaning, and lubricating the unit. [Brown, p31]

81 **b** Sections that are thicker than 5-6 μm in thickness will show overlapping nuclei. [Carson & Cappellano, p59]

82 **b** Immunofluorescence and enzyme histochemical studies are primarily done on unfixed frozen sections. [Brown, p27]

83 **d** When the cortex of a femoral head section shatters, it is most likely underdecalcified. [Carson & Cappellano, pp48-49]

84 **c** Fingernails are hard keratin, so facing the block and soaking it in a solution that softens keratin should help in obtaining a good section. [Bancroft & Gamble, p96; Young & Lowe, p170]

85 **c** When too much water remains under the mounted section when the slide is placed in a hot dryer, nuclear bubbling may result; slides should always be allowed to drain before drying. [Brown, p8]

86 **d** The Histology Quality Improvement Program (HQIP) found that the most common microtomy problem in the first 8 challenges were wrinkles and folds, with an average of 30% of the slides showing this artifact. [Brown, p16]

87 **a** When sections are incompletely fixed and/or processed, they tend to fragment, tear, or disintegrate in the flotation bath. [Brown, p17]

88 **c** Coolant sprays used on a block during microtome may cause cracking of the block, which will result in a parched earth appearance in the section. [Brown, p23]

89 **b** The very serious microtomy artifact in the histopathology laboratory is the carryover of tissue from one case to another slide; the flotation bath should have the surface skimmed between blocks or cases. [Carson & Cappellano, p74]

90 **c** The tissue has most likely been overdehydrated and soaking the faced block with moistened cotton will most likely improve sectioning. [Carson & Cappellano, p64]

The following items (*) have been identified as more appropriate for entry level histotechnologists.

*91 **c** Diamond knives are preferred for cutting 90 nm sections of epoxy embedded tissue. [Carson & Cappellano, p41]

*92 **d** Too much, not too little, blade tilt will cause chatter in microscopic sections; all other items listed will also cause chatter. [Carson & Cappellano, p64]

*93 **d** The isopentane should be at −150°C for the best freezing of skeletal muscle tissue; if it is not cold enough the freezing is slower and holes will be seen in the sections. [Carson & Cappellano, p50]

*94 **c** Thick sections for electron microscopy (primarily for orientation by light microscopy) are cut at 0.5 - 1.0 μm. [Carson & Cappellano, p41]

*95 **a** The tissue seen in the image is kidney and for diagnostic purposes should be cut at 2 μm. [Carson & Cappellano, p59]

*96 **c** Too much, not too little, blade tilt will cause chatter in microscopic sections; all other items listed will also cause chatter. [Carson & Cappellano, p64]

*97 **d** Infiltrating fixed tissue with 30% sucrose will greatly improve cryotomy. [Carson & Cappellano, p51]

*98 **a** Cutting too rapidly will cause the artifact seen in the image; one revolution of the handwheel per second is appropriate for paraffin sectioning. [Carson & Cappellano, p64]

*99 **c** The isopentane should be at –150°C for the best freezing of skeletal muscle tissue; if it is not cold enough the freezing is slower and holes will be seen in the sections. [Carson & Cappellano, p50]

*100 **d** Rocking the handwheel of the microtome while sectioning is a bad practice and may lead to carpal tunnel syndrome. The entire arm should be used to make complete revolutions of the handwheel when sectioning with a nonautomated microtome. [Carson & Cappellano, p88]

*101 **c** Naphthol AS-D chloroacetate esterase stains are rare among the enzyme techniques because paraffin sections of any well fixed tissue may be used. Sections of bone may be used provided decalcification was done with EDTA. [Carson & Cappellano, p302]

*102 **c** The image shown is a Luxol fast blue stain for myelin, and sections should be cut at 10 – 15 μm. [Carson & Cappellano, p206]

*103 **a** Grit or dirt in the plastic block will cause scratches in the section. If the block must be sectioned, an old knife should be used. [Bancroft & Gamble, p613]

*104 **d** The ultramicrotome is used for sectioning for the electron microscope. [Carson & Cappellano, p58]

*105 **d** Enzyme stains are commonly done on muscle biopsies to distinguish between myopathic and neuropathic disease processes. For an accurate diagnosis, multiple enzyme stains are commonly done, frozen sections for these stains should be cut at 8 - 10 μm. [Bancroft & Gamble, p423; Carson & Cappellano, pp294, 301]

*106 **c** The square object is a 2D bar code that allows more information to be on the label. Such information may include, eg, the patient number, specimen type. [Carson & Cappellano, pp27,333-334]

*107 **d** Ribbons should be stretched gently as they are placed on the flotation bath, and small folds or wrinkles quickly teased out of the section. [Carson & Cappellano, p72]

*108 **a** Glass knives rapidly lose their edge, so should be broken as needed. [Bancroft & Gamble, p609]

*109 **c** Alternate thick and thin sections usually result from either the block, knife, or block holder not tightly clamped. [Carson & Cappellano, p64]

*110 **b** The sliding microtome is used for sectioning celloidin and large paraffin blocks. [Carson & Cappellano, p58]

*111 **b** Plus, or positively charged, slides are manufactured as described. [Bancroft & Gamble, p95]

*112 **d** Glass knives are used for cutting sections of plastic-embedded material; Ralph knives are used to section glycol methacrylate-embedded material, and glass knives are also used for sectioning epoxy resin embedded material for electron microscopy. [Carson & Cappellano, p58]

*113 **d** The stain shown is a polarized Congo red stain of amyloid. For the proper green birefringence as seen, sections should be 8 - 10 μm thick; thinner sections will show red birefringence and thicker section will show yellow birefringence. [Carson & Cappellano, p155]

*114 **c** Since all new instruments must be validated before being put into use, there is no need to consider it when purchasing the instrument. The others should be considered when purchasing new instrumentation. [Carson & Cappellano, p80]

*115 **b** Plastics, such as glycol methacrylate, provide an excellent support for very hard tissue such as undecalcified bone, and it allows 1 - 2 μm sections to be cut. [Carson & Cappellano, p41]

*116 **a** Side-by-side comparisons are a part of the validation process that must be done before new instruments are put into use. The other consideration are a part of the verification process. [Carson & Cappellano, p80]

*117 **a** Paraffin with a melting point of 62°C will be difficult to ribbon; as the melting point increases so does ribboning difficulty. Paraffin with a lower melting point should be ordered and put into use. [Carson & Cappellano, p37]

*118 **c** Flotation baths should be cleaned thoroughly at the end of each day and left to dry overnight, or section contamination may occur. [Carson & Cappellano, p73]

*119 **a** Kidney sections should be cut at 2 to 3 μm for diagnostic evaluation, which usually includes PAMS stained sections. [Carson & Cappellano, pp52, 180-181]

*120 **d** Poor sectioning technique, such as aggressive facing of the block, will cause holes in the sections. [Carson & Cappellano, p61]

*121 **c** Glass knives must be used for obtaining good thin sections of glycol methacrylate embedded tissue. [Carson & Cappellano, p40]

*122 **d** Any damage in the edge of the anti-roll plate will cause a problems with sectioning, such as catch on an area of the plate. [Bancroft & Gamble, p100]

ISBN 978-089189-6494   ©ASCP 2016

*123 **b** The metachromasia of amyloid stained with crystal violet stain will be much more prominent if the sections are cut at 10 - 12 μm. [Carson & Cappellano, p156]

*124 **d** The most appropriate action at this point, if the tissue allows, is to cut and discard ribbons until the holes disappear. [Carson & Cappellano, p62]

*125 **c** Not flattening the tissue during embedding, taking microtomy sections too early, and taking microtomy sections after tissue has been cut away could all cause the incomplete section of the upper piece of tissue. The tissue does not display any cutting artifacts due to blade defects. [Brown, p21; Carson & Cappellano, pp42-43]

*126 **b** The section shows cell shrinkage as demonstrated by the lamina propria pulling apart from the epithelium, and artifactual spaces in the lamina propria. This is most likely caused by not draining water from the slide before placing in a hot dryer. [Brown, p24]

*127 **a** Slides should be allowed to drain for several minutes before drying as close to the melting point of the paraffin as possible. [Carson & Cappellano, pp76]

*128 **c** Congo red stained sections that are too thin show a faint red birefringence; therefore, the microtomists are probably cutting the sections at the routine 4-5 μm. [Carson & Cappellano, pp154-155]

*129 **a** The holes seen in the cryostat section of brain tissue are ice crystal artifacts caused by slow freezing of the tissue; more rapid freezing will prevent this artifact. [Carson & Cappellano, pp50-51]

*130 **c** Nuclear bubbling artifact may result from all of the causes listed except overnight drying of the slides. [Brown, p8]

*131 **b** The carryover of tissue from another block indicates that the flotation bath was not cleaned between blocks, or between different cases. [Brown, p22]

*132 **c** Allowing the flotation bath water to sit overnight before use will allow trapped air to escape. [Brown, p22]

*133 **a** The microtomist is most likely picking up sections too early. Other possible causes not listed are cutting too deep in the block and not flattening the tissue properly during embedding. [Brown, p21]

*134 **b** Although the flotation bath was considered to be the source of tissue floater contaminants in the past, more recently the "dip and dunk" stainers have been identified as the major source of floater contaminants. A major global, multilaboratory study identified an average of 2.34% contaminated slides per laboratory and 250.2 tissue fragments in the reagent baths. [Carson & Cappellano, p69]

ISBN 978-089189-6494 ©ASCP 2016

Staining

The following items have been identified as appropriate for both entry level histotechnicians and histotechnologists.

1   When using the Fite procedure, mycobacteria are stained:

   a blue
   b orange
   c red
   d green

2   Which of the following will bind to acid mucosubstances, which can then be demonstrated by the Prussian blue reaction?

   a diastase
   b dimedone
   c colloidal iron
   d hyaluronidase

3   Duplicate sections are stained with PAS, one with and one without diastase digestion. When the staining results are evaluated, the digested section demonstrates:

   a acid mucosubstances
   b the viability of the Schiff reagent
   c sites where glycogen was removed
   d areas of nonspecific PAS positive staining

4   Which of the following pigments is birefringent?

   a formalin
   b bile
   c lipofuscin
   d melanin

5   Acid mucosubstances and neutral mucosubstances can be differentiated by staining with both:

   a mucicarmine and Weigert iron hematoxylin
   b alcian blue and PAS
   c toluidine blue and aldehyde fuchsin
   d Sudan black and Best carmine

6   In the colloidal iron method of staining, the principle of the reaction is believed
     to be the formation of an ionic bond between ferric iron and the carboxyl and
     sulfate groups of:

     a glycogen
     b lipoproteins
     c neutral mucins
     d acid mucosubstances

7   The technique shown below demonstrates:

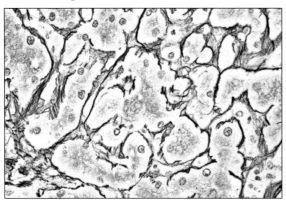

     a basement membranes
     b elastic fibers
     c reducing substances
     d reticulin

8   In order to suppress background and nonspecific staining, a Congo red solution
     frequently contains:

     a sodium acetate
     b sodium chloride
     c sodium phosphate
     d sodium sulfate

9   Acid mucosubstances stained with thionine or azure A exhibit a phenomenon
     known as:

     a orthochromasia
     b polychromasia
     c achromasia
     d metachromasia

10   The PAS reaction is useful for the demonstration of:

     a hyaluronic acid
     b dermatan sulfate
     c chondroitin sulfate B
     d neutral mucosubstances

11 A section of a muscular artery has been stained with the Verhoeff-van Gieson procedure. Microscopic examination shows blue-black nuclei, black elastic fibers, and orange collagen and muscle. The significance of these results is that the:

    a section was overstained in iron hematoxylin
    b staining in van Gieson solution was prolonged
    c picric acid was too dilute
    d stain results are as expected

12 A lymph node is stained with a silver method for reticulin and counterstained with nuclear fast red. After dehydration, there is a film over the entire slide that remains through clearing and coverslipping. The most likely cause is that the:

    a unreacted silver remained on the slide
    b nuclear fast red solution was too concentrated
    c silver solution was contaminated by metal forceps
    d slides were not rinsed with water after counterstaining

13 The black stained structures demonstrated in the image below are most likely:

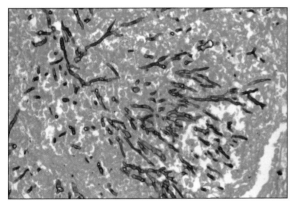

    a calcium
    b fungi
    c urates
    d melanin

14 Yellow-brown pigment, often found in cardiac muscle and liver cells in increasing amounts with age or debilitated states, is known as:

    a porphyrin
    b hemoglobin
    c lipofuscin
    d melanin

15 Hemosiderin, hemoglobin, and bile pigment are classified as:

    a endogenous pigments
    b artifact pigments
    c exogenous pigments
    d extraneous pigments

16 The most appropriate hematoxylin solution for nuclear staining in a lengthy procedure that uses several very acidic solutions is one that is mordanted with:

   a aluminum
   b iron
   c iodine
   d tungsten

17 What micrometer thickness is preferred for the technique shown in below?

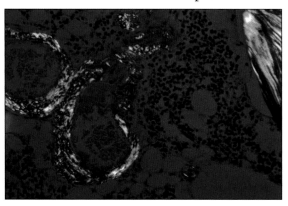

   a 2 to 3
   b 4 to 6
   c 8 to 10
   d 12 to 15

18 A modified phosphotungstic acid-hematoxylin procedure can be used to demonstrate:

   a endothelial cells
   b glial fibers
   c Nissl substance
   d Schwann cells

19 Which of the following is an argyrophil method?

   a Fontana-Masson
   b Gomori-Burtner
   c Grimelius
   d Weigert iron hematoxylin

20 In the Bodian technique, interference with primary staining may occur with prolonged treatment in:

   a sodium thiosulfate
   b oxalic acid
   c gold chloride
   d alcohol

21   The staining intensity of eosin is increased in muscle and red blood cells when tissues are fixed in:

    a 10% neutral buffered formalin
    b Zenker solution
    c Carnoy solution
    d Zamboni PAF solution

22   The laboratory has used all of the supply of aluminum hematoxylin solution. In order to prepare a new solution for immediate use, the solution must be:

    a prepared from hematein
    b air- and light-ripened
    c chemically oxidized
    d made in a small quantity

23   A commonly used connective tissue procedure seen below is the:

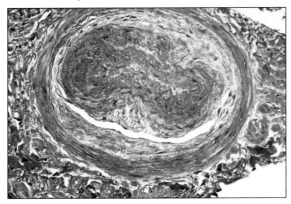

    a Masson trichrome
    b van Gieson
    c Movat pentachrome
    d aldehyde fuchsin

24   When using the cresyl echt violet method, Nissl substance and nuclei can be preferentially stained by varying the degree of differentiation and the:

    a alcohol concentration
    b dye concentration
    c staining time
    d solution pH

25   Muscle that histologically contains cytoplasmic cross-striations and has multiple nuclei located at the edge of the fibers is classified as:

    a smooth
    b visceral
    c skeletal
    d cardiac

26   The method for differentially demonstrating nucleic acids seen below is the:

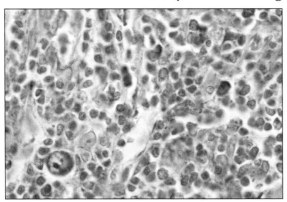

    a Feulgen reaction
    b methyl green-pyronin
    c Masson trichrome
    d Gomori trichrome

27   An effective counterstain following some silver impregnation procedures is:

    a acid fuchsin
    b ethyl green
    c picric acid
    d light green

28   The Fontana-Masson technique may be used to stain:

    a lipids
    b collagen
    c melanin
    d spirochetes

29   Which of the following is a regressive staining method for demonstrating a connective tissue component?

    a Verhoeff-van Gieson
    b Mallory aniline blue
    c Masson trichrome
    d Wilder reticulin

30   The differentiating solution in the Holzer method for glial fibers is:

    a borax ferricyanide
    b alcohol-acetone
    c aniline oil-chloroform
    d alcohol-dioxane

31 The technique shown below is most likely the:

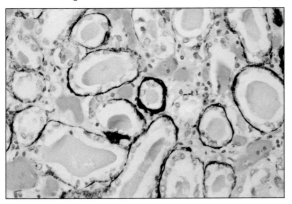

   a Schmorl
   b Grocott
   c Steiner
   d von Kossa

32 Which of the following staining procedures is preferred for demonstrating intracytoplasmic DNA-type viral inclusions in tissue?

   a phloxine-methylene blue
   b Feulgen
   c PTAH
   d Warthin-Starry

33 A solvent that is commonly used in oil red O and Sudan black B solutions to prevent the loss of lipids during fat staining is:

   a xylene
   b 70% ethanol
   c acetone-ethanol
   d propylene glycol

34 In the Verhoeff-van Gieson technique for demonstrating elastic fibers, the Verhoeff staining solution should be used for a only few:

   a hours
   b days
   c weeks
   d months

35 A Ziehl-Neelsen procedure is done on a lung granuloma, but no acid-fast organisms are demonstrated. It would be wise to verify the absence of these organisms by using which of the following procedures?

   a Grocott methenamine silver
   b Truant auramine-rhodamine
   c Warthin-Starry
   d Gram

36 Microscopic inspection of a PAS stained control section for fungi reveals very palely stained fungal organisms, making identification difficult. A likely cause for this problem is the:

     a use of depleted Schiff reagent
     b use of diluted chromic acid solution
     c use of an incorrect reducing agent
     d omission of sodium metabisulfite

37 Unless the methyl green-pyronin procedure has been modified for formalin fixed tissue, which of the following fixatives will give the BEST results with this stain?

     a Bouin
     b Carnoy
     c Zenker
     d Zamboni

38 Examples of natural dyes are:

     a hematoxylin, orcein, and methylene blue
     b aniline blue, carmine, and hematoxylin
     c crystal violet, methyl green, and indigo
     d hematoxylin, carmine, and orcein

39 A chemical that will bleach melanin is:

     a oxalic acid
     b potassium permanganate
     c hydroquinone
     d sodium thiosulfate

40 Which of the following characteristics of ammoniacal silver solutions may cause tissue sections to wash off during impregnation?

     a osmotic pressure
     b alkalinity
     c concentration
     d temperature

41 The primary staining solution used in the Schmorl technique contains ferric chloride and potassium:

     a dichromate
     b iodide
     c ferricyanide
     d ferrocyanide

42   What is the preferred fixative for the stain shown below?

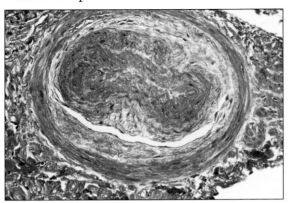

    a   Orth solution
    b   Bouin solution
    c   neutral buffered formalin
    d   glyoxal

43   The primary staining solution for the technique shown on a section of aorta in the image below is:

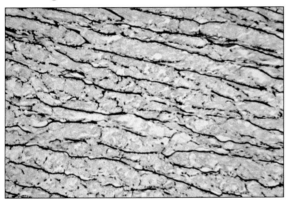

    a   made fresh before each use
    b   aged before use
    c   satisfactory for use indefinitely
    d   satisfactory for use up to one month

44   Microscopic review of a section stained with the Warthin-Starry technique shows the spirochetes stained yellow. The most likely cause of this problem is:

    a   overoxidizing
    b   underdeveloping
    c   dirty glassware
    d   heated impregnating solution

45 Argentaffin cells found in the epithelium of the stomach and intestines are known as which of the following cells?

 a amphophilic
 b enterochromaffin
 c absorptive
 d Paneth

46 Which of the following is used in acid-fast staining procedures to enhance staining and aid in dissolving the fuchsin dye?

 a hydrochloric acid
 b methylene blue
 c phenol
 d water

47 True epithelial cells lining ventricles and the spinal canal are called:

 a astrocytes
 b oligodendroglia
 c microglia
 d ependymal

48 Solutions of anionic dyes in picric acid are used to demonstrate:

 a reticulin
 b fibrocartilage
 c collagen
 d elastin

49 Which of the following pigments can be stained with Sudan black B and carbol fuchsin?

 a bilirubin
 b hemoglobin
 c lipofuscin
 d melanin

50 Transitional epithelium refers to:

 a endothelium
 b urothelium
 c mesothelium
 d metaplasia

51   The substance stained rose-red in the image below is most likely:

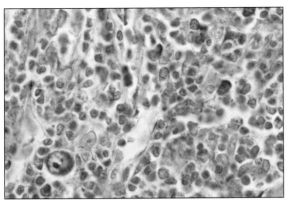

    a mitochondria
    b lysosomes
    c deoxyribonucleic acid
    d ribonucleic acid

52   Which of the following elastic stains performs well after any fixative, gives intense black staining of coarse fibers, must be differentiated microscopically, and gives permanent results with little fading?

    a PTAH
    b Verhoeff
    c Weigert
    d Masson

53   The material stained blue in the image below is:

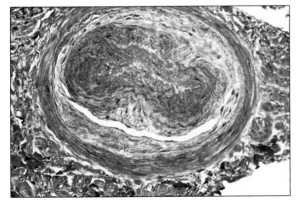

    a cartilage
    b muscle
    c collagen
    d reticulin

54   A technique that can be used to demonstrate lipids in paraffin sections is:

    a staining with Sudan IV
    b fixation with osmium tetroxide
    c fixation with potassium dichromate
    d staining with alizarin red S

55   The reducing agent in diamine silver procedures for reticulin demonstration is most frequently:

    a formaldehyde
    b hydroquinone
    c pyridine
    d pyrogallol

56   The basic component of the central nervous system is the:

    a axon
    b neuron
    c dendrite
    d ganglion

57   Which of the following combination of stains will demonstrate both the myelin sheath and nerve fibers?

    a gallocyanine and Bodian
    b Nonidez and Bielschowsky
    c Luxol fast blue and Holmes
    d Sevier-Munger and thionin

58   The technique shown in the image below is the:

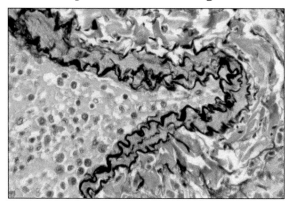

    a Hotchkiss-McManus
    b Grocott methenamine silver
    c Verhoeff-van Gieson
    d von Kossa

59 The most consistently reliable technique for demonstrating fungi in tissues is the:

   a Gridley
   b Brown and Brenn
   c Grocott methenamine silver
   d Ziehl-Neelsen

60 In addition to hematoxylin and potassium or ammonium alum, a traditional solution of Mayer hematoxylin contains:

   a 95% alcohol and glycerol
   b 95% alcohol, glycerol, and acetic acid
   c sodium iodate, chloral hydrate, and acetic acid
   d sodium iodate, chloral hydrate and citric acid

61 For light microscopic evaluation it is generally necessary to use special stains to demonstrate fungi in tissue sections because most fungi:

   a can only be seen using silver impregnation
   b are removed in the routine staining process
   c stain only after reduction of polysaccharides
   d are inconspicuous with the H&E procedure

62 Which of the following staining procedures is most suitable for demonstrating general tissue morphology?

   a periodic acid-Schiff
   b Verhoeff-van Gieson
   c hematoxylin and eosin
   d Wilder reticulin

63 An example of an exogenous pigment is:

   a argentaffin
   b melanin
   c chromaffin
   d carbon

64 The sequence of reactions in the Wilder and Snook ammoniacal silver methods for demonstrating reticulin fibers is:

   a sensitization, oxidation, silver impregnation, reduction
   b oxidation, sensitization, silver impregnation, reduction
   c oxidation, sensitization, reduction, silver impregnation
   d sensitization, silver impregnation, oxidation, reduction

65   The technique shown below demonstrates:

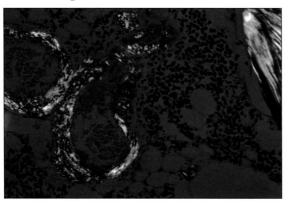

   a birefringence
   b dichroism
   c fluorescence
   d phase contrast

66   The largest portion of the brain is the:

   a medulla
   b midbrain
   c cerebellum
   d cerebrum

67   Hemosiderin-laden macrophages present in the alveolar spaces of the lung can be distinguished from other pigmented macrophages by the following reagent/ reaction:

   a Prussian blue
   b Fouchet
   c silver nitrate
   d azocarmine B

68   The pigment commonly known as "wear and tear pigment" or "brown atrophy" is:

   a hemofuchsin
   b ceroid
   c lipofuscin
   d hemosiderin

69   To properly classify bone, it may be described as:

   a glial and astrocytic
   b cancellous and compact
   c smooth and striated
   d ground substance

70 Melanin is normally found in the:

   a kidney
   b liver
   c skin
   d stomach

71 A Gram stain has been done on a reactive, inflammatory lymph node, and the background structures are stained intense red, making identification of Gram negative organisms very difficult. This is most likely due to:

   a prolonged staining with basic fuchsin
   b drying following the crystal violet
   c poor differentiation with picric acid-acetone
   d incomplete dehydration and clearing

72 Which of the following acids in an alcoholic solution is most commonly used to differentiate aluminum-hematoxylin stained sections?

   a formic
   b hydrochloric
   c sulfuric
   d acetic

73 The material stained purple in the large cells is:

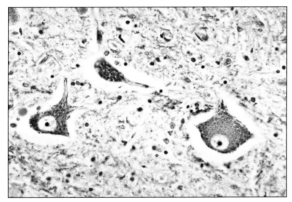

   a euchromatin
   b lipofuscin
   c chromaffin granules
   d Nissl substance

74 Which of the following is a metachromatic stain used for identifying mast cells?

   a aniline blue
   b Luxol fast blue
   c toluidine blue
   d Giemsa

75 Connective tissue proper refers to tissue composed of:

   a spongy, cancellous, and cortical bone
   b hyaline and fibrocartilage
   c hematopoietic bone marrow
   d collagen, reticulin, and elastin

76 The fibers stained purple in the image below are:

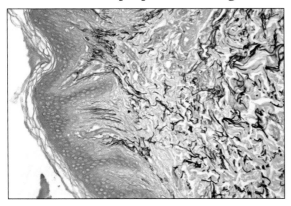

   a reticulin
   b collagen
   c elastic
   d plasmalemma

77 The purpose of iodine in Gram procedures for staining bacteria is to:

   a make the cell walls of bacteria permeable
   b form a dye-complex with crystal violet
   c decolorize crystal violet
   d inactivate bacteria

78 The terms "squamous," "cuboidal," and "columnar" describe cells of which tissue type?

   a connective
   b muscle
   c epithelial
   d bone

79 The atomic grouping within a dye that gives it its color is called a/an:

   a chromophore
   b chromogen
   c auxochrome
   d lake

80   In which of the following staining methods for nerve fibers is hydroquinone used?

     a   Mallory
     b   Weil
     c   Bodian
     d   Holzer

81   The stain shown below is most likely the :

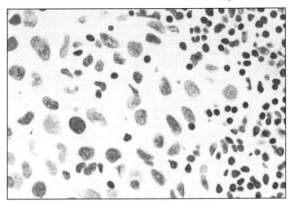

     a   PAS
     b   methyl green-pyronin
     c   cresyl echt violet
     d   Feulgen

82   Bacteria stain either Gram-positive or Gram-negative due to differences in:

     a   shape
     b   cell walls
     c   size
     d   location

83   Which of the following chemicals is used as both a mordant and a differentiator in the Weil stain for myelin?

     a   mercuric chloride
     b   chromium aluminum sulfate
     c   aluminum ammonium sulfate
     d   ferric ammonium sulfate

84   Fixation of tissues for 2 weeks in which of the following will most likely impair nuclear basophilia?

     a   neutral buffered formalin
     b   Zenker solution
     c   paraformaldehyde
     d   glyoxal

85 A researcher wishes to differentiate the different types of granulocytes in a tissue section. The stain of choice is:

a Gram
b acid-fast
c Romanowsky
d silver impregnation

86 A substance that has the ability to both bind silver and reduce it to a visible metallic form is said to be:

a argyrophilic
b argentaffin
c amphophilic
d auxochromic

87 After H&E staining, the cytoplasm in a tissue section appears hazy, obscure, and contrasts poorly with the nuclei. The most likely cause is that:

a eosin Y was used
b phloxine was added to the eosin
c acetic acid was present in the eosin solution
d slides were not adequately dehydrated

88 The cells stained blue in the tissue shown below are:

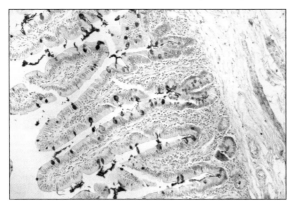

a goblet
b Paneth
c argentaffin
d chromaffin

89 Microscopic review of auramine-rhodamine stained control slides will reveal:

a fungal organisms
b yeast forms
c mycobacteria
d spirochetes

90   When the auxochrome of a dye is the COOH group, the dye is:

    a anionic
    b cationic
    c amphoteric
    d polychromatic

91   The Stein and Hall techniques are based on the conversion of bile pigment to:

    a porphyrins
    b biliverdin
    c hemoglobin
    d aposiderin

92   The acid used in the Prussian blue reaction is:

    a acetic
    b hydrochloric
    c nitric
    d sulfuric

93   The structures stained blue-black in the image below are:

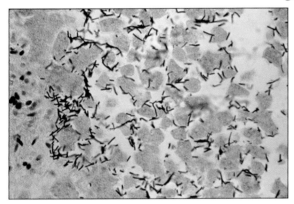

    a Gram positive
    b Gram negative
    c acid-fast
    d argentaffin

94   Areolar connective tissue is also known as:

    a mineralized connective tissue
    b dense connective tissue
    c loose connective tissue
    d specialized connective tissue

95   A hematoxylin solution that is ONLY used progressively is:

    a Harris
    b Ehrlich
    c Mayer
    d Delafield

96   Nuclei stained with hematoxylin are predominately red-brown to red. This is most
      likely because of the use of:

      a insufficient differentiation
      b prolonged neutralization
      c a nonacidified hematoxylin solution
      d overoxidized hematoxylin

97   In the Hall method, Fouchet reagent is used to demonstrate:

      a copper
      b bile
      c lipofuscin
      d melanin

98   To achieve the desired intensity of purple when using the Gomori aldehyde
      fuchsin stain for demonstrating elastic tissue, the paraldehyde used to prepare
      the reagent should be:

      a aged
      b fresh
      c chilled
      d heated

99   A problem will occur in the stain illustrated below if the:

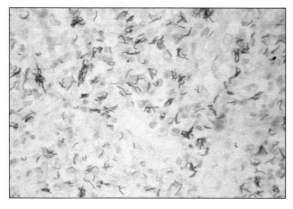

      a sections dry after the carbol-fuchsin
      b carbol-fuchsin is prepared from pararosaniline
      c acid-alcohol is removed with tap-water
      d carbol-fuchsin contains a wetting agent

100   Microscopic examination of an H&E stained section shows a pink artifact
      surrounding the tissue and in tissue spaces. The most probable cause of this
      artifact is:

      a precipitation of the eosin
      b excess acetic acid in the eosin
      c surplus adhesive on the slide
      d poor bluing of the hematoxylin

101 In the Mallory phosphotungstic acid-hematoxylin (PTAH) method, skeletal muscle striations stain:

   a blue
   b red
   c black
   d yellow

102 Acidophilic tissue components that should appear stained different shades of pink following H&E staining are:

   a muscle, collagen, and erythrocytes
   b muscle, reticulin, and elastin
   c collagen, basement membrane, and nucleic acids

103 In order for the Gram stain to work properly, it is important to apply the mordant:

   a after the crystal violet
   b prior to any of the stains
   c combined with the primary dye
   d after the counterstain

104 Which of the following methods use a methenamine solution?

   a Foot-Bielschowsky and Bodian
   b Wilder and Snook
   c Gomori and Grocott
   d Gridley-Laidlaw

105 The tissue shown in the image below is:

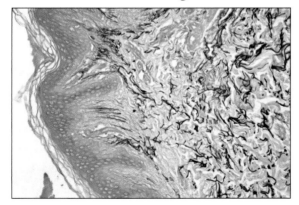

   a tonsil
   b cervix
   c esophagus
   d skin

106 Differential staining of nuclei and cytoplasm with Giemsa solution is an example of:

    a polychromasia
    b metachromasia
    c orthochromasia
    d hypochromasia

107 Which of the following histologic features is unique to cardiac muscle?

    a cross-striations
    b peripherally located nuclei
    c intercalated discs
    d nonbranching fibers

108 Pigment that is present on the surface of cells but NOT within them is probably:

    a endogenous
    b hematogenous
    c hepatogenous
    d artifactual

109 Oligodendroglia are cells that function in the production and maintenance of myelin sheaths that surround:

    a axons
    b neuroglia
    c microglia
    d astrocytes

110 Which of the following is an example of a metachromatic stain?

    a Congo red
    b orange G
    c toluidine blue
    d thioflavin T

111 The primary stain used in the technique shown below is:

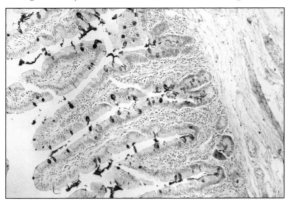

    a methylene blue
    b Prussian blue
    c colloidal iron
    d iron hematoxylin

112 Which of the following procedures will demonstrate most amoebae in tissue sections?

    a Grocott methenamine silver
    b Kinyoun acid-fast
    c Mayer mucicarmine
    d periodic acid-Schiff

113 Which of the following is an iron hematoxylin solution that is frequently used for nuclear staining?

    a Harris
    b Delafield
    c Mayer
    d Weigert

114 The pigment that is formed following a reaction of ferrous ions with potassium ferricyanide is known as:

    a Prussian blue
    b methylene blue
    c Turnbull blue
    d Nile blue

115 The stain shown below is NOT an excellent hematoxylin and eosin because:

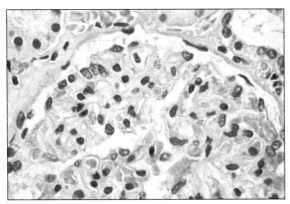

    a only 2 shades of eosin are apparent
    b various chromatin patterns cannot be seen
    c the hematoxylin is breaking down
    d red cells are not identifiable

116 The stain procedure that produces a red-orange result for calcium deposits in tissue is:

    a von Kossa
    b alizarin red S
    c Kinyoun
    d Mayer mucicarmine

117 Connective tissue cells that have many cytoplasmic granules that stain metachromatically are:

    a Purkinje cells
    b macrophages
    c enterochromaffin cells
    d mast cells

118 The green stained substance shown below is most likely:

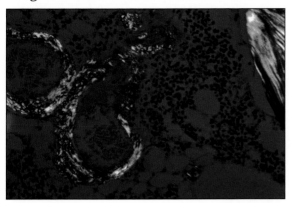

   a collagen
   b elastic tissue
   c smooth muscle
   d amyloid

119 Stains for simple lipids are performed on which of the following sections:

   a paraffin
   b frozen
   c celloidin
   d glycol methacrylate

120 The toughest of the connective tissue fibers is:

   a reticulin
   b elastin
   c collagen
   d myelin

121 Which of the following is the ONLY hematogenous pigment found in normal red blood cells?

   a hemoglobin
   b hemosiderin
   c hematoidin
   d hemozoon

122 Oil red O staining is based on the principle of:

   a impregnation
   b birefringence
   c ionic linkages
   d absorption

123 Which of the following methods involves the reduction of ferric ions to ferrous ions followed by precipitation with the Turnbull blue reaction?

  a Schmorl
  b Grimelius
  c Sevier-Munger
  d Gmelin

124 The tissue shown in the image below is:

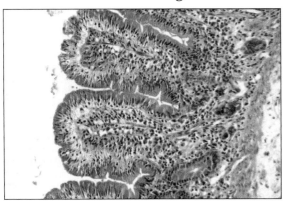

  a esophagus
  b stomach
  c small intestine
  d colon

125 In the Gomori aldehyde fuchsin technique, elastic fibers stain:

  a blue to black
  b violet-purple
  c reddish-brown
  d bluish-green

126 Urate crystals can be demonstrated with:

  a rubeanic acid
  b leucofuchsin
  c methenamine silver
  d aldehyde fuchsin

127 A method that will selectively stain astrocytes in frozen sections is the:

  a Cajal gold sublimate
  b Sevier-Munger
  c Pal-Weigert
  d Mallory PTAH

128 Which of the following is an argyrophil stain that will demonstrate both neurofibrils and neurosecretory granules?

   a Cajal
   b Fontana-Masson
   c Sevier-Munger
   d Weil

129 Some argentaffin cells are also known as:

   a Kupffer cells
   b Grimelius cells
   c Paneth cells
   d Kulchitsky cells

130 The staining pattern seen in the image below is typically seen in tissue from the:

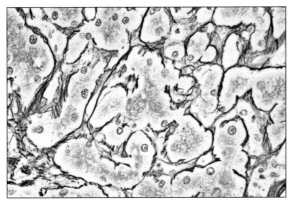

   a pancreas
   b lymph node
   c kidney
   d liver

131 Which of the following acts as the differentiating solution in the Verhoeff-van Gieson procedure?

   a Weigert iodine solution
   b borax ferricyanide
   c ferric chloride
   d acid alcohol

132 The staining mechanism in which metallic substances are selectively deposited on structures and made visible by reduction of the metal is called:

   a substantive
   b adjective
   c progressive
   d impregnation

133   *Entamoeba histolytica* can be demonstrated with which of the following procedures or methods?

     a   Gordon-Sweets
     b   von Kossa
     c   periodic acid-Schiff
     d   Schmorl

134   In the Gomori 1-step trichrome stain, collagen stains:

     a   yellow
     b   green
     c   black
     d   red

135   In humans, nonkeratinizing stratified squamous epithelium is found covering/lining the:

     a   skin
     b   trachea
     c   esophagus
     d   urinary bladder

136   The cytoplasmic granules in connective tissue mast cells stain well with:

     a   toluidine blue
     b   eosin
     c   phloxine
     d   orange G

137   The counterstain for the procedure shown below contains:

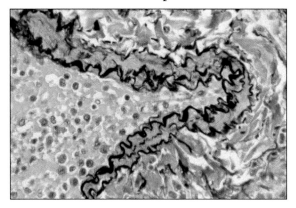

     a   metanil yellow
     b   basic fuchsin
     c   picric acid
     d   orange G

138 Granules found in cells of the adrenal medulla that are preserved only when fixed in Orth solution are called:

  a melanin
  b lipofuscin
  c chromaffin
  d chromatin

139 The organisms stained red in the image below are:

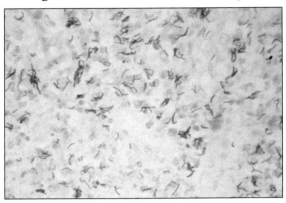

  a rickettsia
  b mycobacteria
  c chlamydiae
  d filamentous fungi

140 Microscopic examination of an H&E stained brain section reveals basophilic material in the cytoplasm of the neurons. This material is most likely:

  a secretory granules
  b neurofilaments
  c RNA
  d lipids

141 Which of the following methods is a modification of the Bodian technique that uses a buffered impregnating solution to increase the specificity of the stain?

  a Rio-Hortega
  b Nonidez
  c Bielschowsky
  d Holmes

142 Which of the following stains is dependent upon differences in the bacterial cell wall for differential staining?

  a Gridley
  b Gram
  c Grocott
  d Warthin-Starry

143 Acid-alcohol decolorizers are generally recommended over aqueous decolorizers for use with acid-fast procedures because alcoholic solutions:

   a are more stable
   b begin dehydration
   c penetrate more slowly
   d allow more uniform decolorization

144 The technique shown below depends upon the:

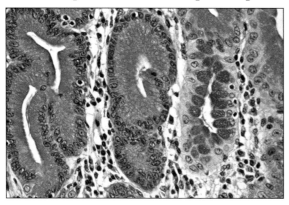

   a formation of aldehydes
   b presence of the carboxylate group
   c presence of the sulfate group
   d digestion with hyaluronidase

145 Which of the following hematoxylin solutions contains ethylene glycol and aluminum sulfate?

   a Harris
   b Delafield
   c Gill
   d Mayer

146 The bacterium *Legionella pneumophila* can be demonstrated using which staining method?

   a Schleifstein
   b Pinkerton
   c May-Grunwald
   d Steiner

147 In the Jones and Gomori methenamine silver techniques for basement membranes, sections are oxidized with:

   a potassium permanganate
   b chromic acid
   c lithium carbonate
   d periodic acid

148 False positive results may occur with the technique shown below if the tissue is fixed in:

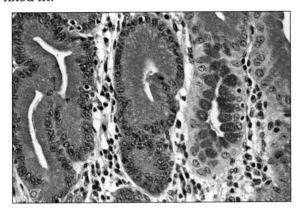

    a glyoxal
    b glutaraldehyde
    c Bouin solution
    d Zenker solution

149 In the technique shown below, formaldehyde is used as a/an:

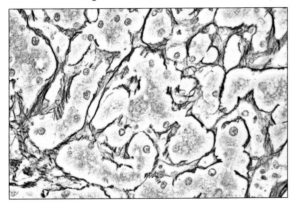

    a reducer
    b sensitizer
    c oxidizer
    d toner

150 Nissl substance can be demonstrated with which of the following stains?

    a thionin and cresyl echt violet
    b eosin and phloxine
    c silver nitrate and gold sublimate
    d orange G and methyl blue

151 The tissue seen below is:

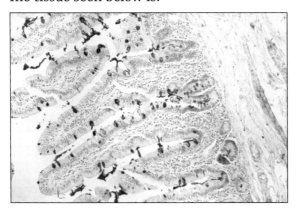

   a esophagus
   b small intestine
   c appendix
   d colon

152 In the Wilder technique for demonstrating reticulin, uranyl nitrate acts as a(n):

   a mordant
   b accentuator
   c sensitizer
   d toner

153 Microscopic evaluation of an H&E stained section reveals dark deposits of material dispersed irregularly over the tissue. The most likely cause of this problem is that the hematoxylin solution:

   a was not filtered before use
   b is past its useful shelf life
   c contains too much acetic acid
   d does not contain an oxidizer

154 Microscopic review of a GMS stained section shows connective tissue fibers and erythrocytes stained black. This is most likely the result of:

   a overexposure to hot methenamine silver
   b underexposure to gold chloride
   c underexposure to sodium thiosulfate
   d performing the procedure in a microwave oven

155 During microscopic examination of a fungus stain, extraneous fungal elements are seen above rather than in the section. The most likely cause for this problem is:

   a poor dehydration prior to coverslipping
   b prolonged exposure to silver solution
   c contaminated staining solutions
   d a bacterial rather than fungal disease

156 Tissue components stained red-orange in the image seen below are:

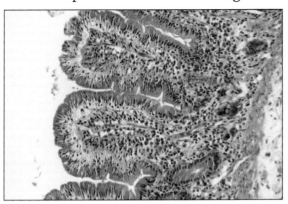

   a Kulchitsky cells
   b Paneth granules
   c lipid droplets
   d goblet cells

157 Sections of lung stained with both the GMS and the PAS show positive staining
     of what appear to be fungal organisms. However, the same oval-shaped bodies are
     seen in nongranulomatous areas and on edges of the tissue. Polarization of the
     bodies reveals a Maltese cross configuration. This "positive" staining material is
     therefore most likely:

   a calcium
   b ceroid
   c talcum powder
   d asbestos

158 Spirochetes are filamentous bacteria that are known to be:

   a argentophilic
   b argyrophilic
   c polychromatic
   d metachromatic

159 Following hematoxylin and eosin staining, slides are dehydrated through
     ascending strengths of alcohol and cleared in xylene; however, the first xylene in
     the series is milky white. The most appropriate action is to:

   a change all solutions
   b change all clearing solutions
   c change all dehydrating and clearing solutions
   d air-dry slides and dehydrate and clear as usual

160 The large cells seen below that contain purple granular material in the cytoplasm are:

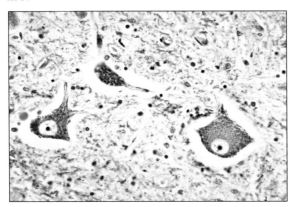

   a astrocytes
   b Purkinje cells
   c neurons
   d plasma cells

161 If hematoxylin is unavailable, which of the following dyes is recommended as a substitute in a routine hematoxylin and eosin procedure?

   a methyl blue
   b aniline blue
   c Nile blue A
   d Celestine blue

162 The phosphotungstic acid-hematoxylin (PTAH) stain is useful for demonstrating:

   a edema fluid
   b muscle striations
   c ground substance
   d reticulin network

163 Hemosiderin is thought to be composed of ferric iron and:

   a protein
   b collagen
   c chromatin
   d fatty acid

164 Whether collagen fibers are found in a dense regular arrangement or in an irregular arrangement varies with the:

   a heredity and sex of the individual
   b location and function
   c size of the organ
   d age of the individual

165 Microscopic review of sections stained with hematoxylin and eosin reveals very pink cytoplasm and pale reddish-brown nuclei. Of the following, the most appropriate action is to:

    a restain the sections for a longer time in hematoxylin
    b discard and replace the ammonia water
    c replace the hematoxylin with solution from another batch
    d change all solutions and restain the sections

166 In silver impregnation techniques, the use of improperly cleaned glassware results in:

    a the absence of silver staining
    b nonselective silver precipitation
    c inadequate counterstaining
    d the inability to tone

167 Which of the following methods stains elastic tissue brown?

    a acid orcein
    b resorcin-fuchsin
    c Gomori aldehyde fuchsin
    d Verhoeff-van Gieson

168 The technique shown below will NOT be satisfactory if the tissue has been fixed in:

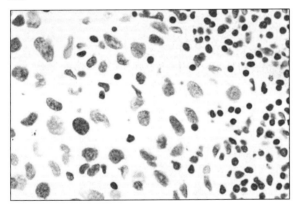

    a Zenker solution
    b Bouin solution
    c zinc formalin
    d glyoxal

169   The preferred control for the technique shown below is:

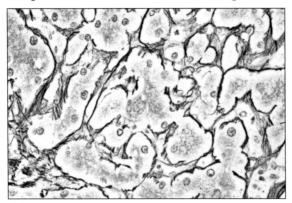

    a pancreas
    b liver
    c kidney
    d uterus

170   The pathologist has requested a Feulgen procedure on a lymph node. The staining sequence for this procedure is:

    a hydrochloric acid, sulfurous acid, Schiff, light green
    b periodic acid, Schiff, sulfurous acid, light green
    c hydrochloric acid, Schiff, sulfurous acid, light green
    d Schiff, hydrochloric acid, light green

171   Fresh silver solutions were properly prepared and used in a Warthin-Starry technique. After completion of the procedure, the positive control does not demonstrate spirochetes. Of the following, the most likely reason for this problem is:

    a poorly fixed tissue
    b contaminated glassware
    c improperly prepared developing solution
    d incorrectly selected mordant

172   The function of Bouin fluid in trichrome stains is that of a/an:

    a mordant
    b reducer
    c oxidizer
    d sensitizer

173   In order to protect the leprosy organism from extraction of the acid-fast component, sections are deparaffinized in xylene and:

    a peanut oil
    b dioxane
    c alcohol
    d acetone

174 Another techniques that can be used to demonstrate the material stained black in the image below is::

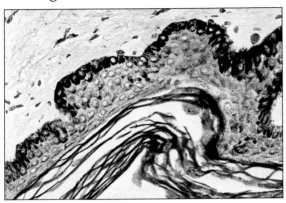

   a Grocott
   b von Kossa
   c Schmorl
   d PAS

175 In the Verhoeff-van Gieson technique, ferric chloride and iodine in the Verhoeff solution function initially as mordants and then as:

   a neutralizers
   b differentiators
   c sensitizers
   d oxidizers

176 A black pigment that is insoluble, often found in the lungs and hilar lymph nodes, cannot be bleached, and cannot be identified by typical chemical reactions for pigments is most likely:

   a hemosiderin
   b melanin
   c lipofuscin
   d anthracotic

177 Which of the following tissue components can be stained by Weigert resorcin-fuchsin, Hart resorcin-fuchsin, or orcein?

   a reticular fibers
   b myosin fibers
   c elastic fibers
   d collagen fibers

178 Sections stained with the Grocott procedure for fungi were originally completely satisfactory. After several weeks of being exposed to light, however, a granular black precipitate can be seen over the sections. This is most likely due to the omission during staining of:

   a chromic acid
   b gold chloride
   c sodium bisulfite
   d sodium thiosulfate

179 The technique illustrated below demonstrates:

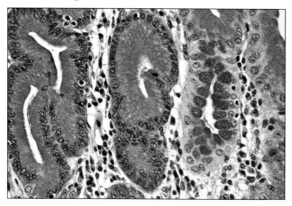

   a sulfated acid mucopolysaccharides
   b carboxylated acid mucopolysaccharides
   c chondroitin sulfate and heparin
   d neutral mucopolysaccharides

180 Mordants for hematoxylin are generally classified as:

   a amphoteric
   b weakly acidic
   c metallic
   d gaseous

181 The oxidizer in the Wilder procedure for reticulin fibers is:

   a potassium permanganate
   b phosphomolybdic acid
   c periodic acid
   d chromic acid

182 The technique shown below is the:

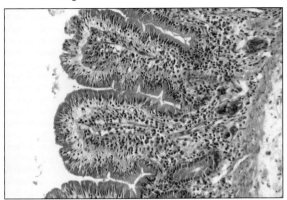

  a Mayer mucicarmine
  b oil red O
  c Congo red
  d alizarin red S

183 The oxidizer used in the Gomori reticulin method is:

  a periodic acid
  b chromic acid
  c potassium permanganate
  d phosphomolybdic acid

184 The purpose of nonmetallic forceps and chemically-cleaned glassware in silver techniques is to prevent:

  a premature uptake of silver
  b changes in pH of the silver solution
  c false negative staining
  d contamination of the silver solution

185 The black stained structures in the image below are most likely:

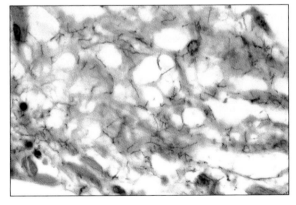

  a mycobacteria
  b staphylococci
  c rickettsia
  d spirochetes

186 Another name for fat cells is:

    a APUD cells
    b myocytes
    c adipocytes
    d histiocytes

187 Elastic fibers have an affinity for which of the following stains?

    a Sudan
    b indigo
    c brazilin
    d orcein

188 Of the following, the most reliable stain for demonstrating Gram negative bacteria in tissue sections is the:

    a Giemsa
    b Brown-Hopps
    c Ziehl-Neelsen
    d Grocott

189 A delicate 3-dimensional connective tissue meshwork that forms the framework of organs such as the spleen and lymph nodes is made of:

    a elastic fibers
    b reticular fibers
    c smooth muscle
    d basement membrane

190 Chromic acid is used in the method shown below to:

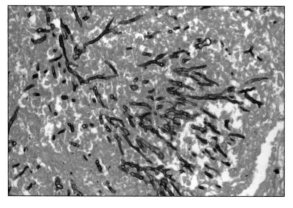

    a prevent overoxidation of weak polysaccharides
    b mordant formaldehyde-fixed tissues
    c oxidize polysaccharides to aldehydes
    d begin impregnation

191 In the Bodian technique, Protargol impregnates both neurofibrils and connective tissue. Subsequently, connective tissue is rendered colorless by replacement of the silver with:

  a copper
  b gold
  c lead
  d tin

192 A term used to designate the disease produced by the organisms shown below is:

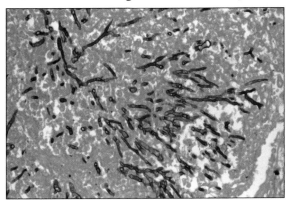

  a inflammation
  b mycosis
  c viral
  d parasitic

193 The primary dye used in a rapid, non-silver staining procedure to demonstrate *Helicobacter pylori* is a/an:

  a azure-eosin
  b leucofuchsin
  c colloidal iron
  d carbol-fuchsin

194 EA solutions used in cytologic staining contain:

  a fast green, eosin Y, and phosphomolybdic acid
  b Orange G, phosphotungstic acid, and eosin Y
  c light green, orange G, and phosphomolybdic acid
  d light green, eosin Y, and phosphotungstic acid

195 With the use of epitope retrieval methods for immunohistochemical staining:

  a more concentrated antibodies are needed
  b antigen detection is improved
  c there is increased background staining
  d less uniform staining is achieved

196   In the Feulgen reaction for nucleic acids, slides are placed in 1N hydrochloric acid to promote:

    a autolysis
    b oxidation
    c hydrolysis
    d anabolism

197   The method shown below uses silver to demonstrate:

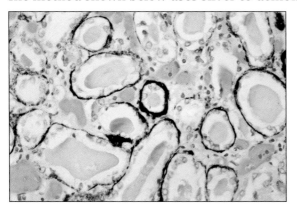

    a calcium
    b phosphates
    c aldehydes
    d urates

198   The Grocott methenamine silver method can be used to demonstrate:

    a urate crystals
    b argyrophilic cells
    c hemosiderin
    d copper

199   Avidin-biotin methods are used in:

    a electron microscopy
    b enzyme histochemistry
    c immunohistochemistry
    d lipid chemistry

200   The Schmorl method will stain reducing substances:

    a blue
    b red
    c black
    d brown

201 The oxidizer used in the technique shown below is:

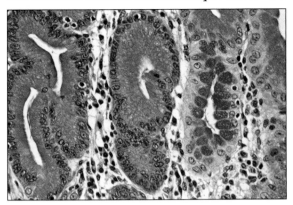

   a chromic acid
   b periodic acid
   c potassium permanganate
   d sodium metabisulfite

202 Microscopic evaluation of a Giemsa stained bone marrow section reveals poor nuclear staining and very little cytoplasmic differentiation. This is most likely the result of:

   a an improper pH
   b sections that are too thin
   c the staining solution that is not ripened
   d staining done at room temperature

203 A component in the cell nucleus that stains strongly with basic dyes is called:

   a endoplasmic reticulum
   b cytomembrane
   c lipofuscin
   d chromatin

204 The nerve process that carries electrical impulses away from the cell body is called a(n):

   a neuron
   b dendrite
   c synapse
   d axon

205 Differentiating agents in the Luxol fast blue procedure for myelin are:

   a sodium borate and potassium ferrocyanide
   b absolute alcohol and aniline oil
   c gold chloride and sodium thiosulfate
   d lithium carbonate and 70% alcohol

206 The blue stained substance shown below is demonstrated in a method using hydrochloric acid and:

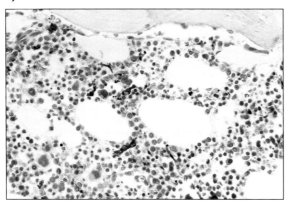

   a colloidal iron
   b potassium ferricyanide
   c potassium ferrocyanide
   d methylene blue

207 In the Masson trichrome method, muscle fibers are colored:

   a red
   b blue
   c yellow
   d green

208 The most sensitive solution for detecting copper in tissue is:

   a chloranilic acid
   b rhodanine
   c orcein
   d aldehyde fuchsin

209 The molecule that produces an immune response in animals is called a/an:

   a antibody
   b antisera
   c immunoglobulin
   d antigen

210 Which of the following chemicals functions as an oxidizer?

   a aluminum sulfate
   b sodium sulfite
   c potassium permanganate
   d acetic acid

211 The structures shown in the technique below stain black with silver because of the:

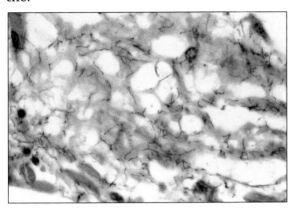

    a subsequent application of a chemical reducing agent
    b inherent ability of the organism to reduce silver
    c specificity of the method for organisms
    d formation of ionic bonds

212 The most commonly used dye solution for staining *Mycobacterium tuberculosis* is composed of:

    a basic fuchsin and phenol
    b acid fuchsin and formalin
    c acid fuchsin and carbolic acid
    d new fuchsin and hydrochloric acid

213 Ammonia water, lithium carbonate solution, and Scott tap water substitute are examples of:

    a decolorizers
    b accentuators
    c differentiators
    d bluing agents

214   The black stained filamentous structures seen below are known as:

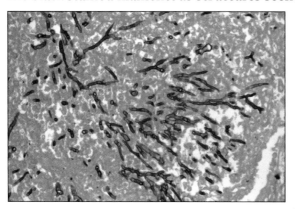

    a yeasts
    b dimorphic
    c septa
    d hyphae

215   The first cytoplasmic stain in the Papanicolaou technique is OG-6 and the second cytoplasmic stain is:

    a metachromatic
    b fluorescent
    c polychromatic
    d argyrophilic

216   In the Brown-Hopps stain, one of the differentiating solutions is:

    a acid alcohol
    b Gram iodine
    c Gallego solution
    d 75% alcohol

217   In the Verhoeff-van Gieson technique, elastic fibers stain:

    a red to purple
    b blue-black to black
    c yellow to brown
    d blue to blue-green

218   The most commonly used chemical for reducing adsorbed silver to a visible metallic state in argyrophil procedures such as the Warthin-Starry is:

    a sodium thiosulfate
    b uranyl nitrate
    c hydroquinone
    d sodium bisulfate

219 The blue-black structures shown in the technique below are most likely:

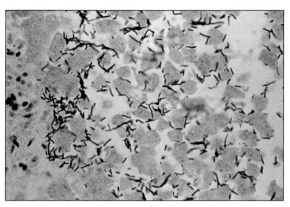

   a mycobacteria
   b spirochetes
   c bacilli
   d hyphae

220 The term "argentaffin" literally denotes a reaction wherein cells have the ability to reduce a salt of:

   a chromium
   b lithium
   c copper
   d silver

221 When excessive melanin deposition interferes with examination of cellular morphology, melanin pigment can be removed by bleaching a section with:

   a sodium thiosulfate
   b hydroquinone
   c potassium permanganate
   d ammoniacal silver

222 The selectivity for nuclear staining by Harris hematoxylin can be increased by adding:

   a aluminum salts
   b sodium iodate
   c glycerol
   d alcohol

223 A stained section mounted with a synthetic resin appears cloudy. This is most likely the result of using a mounting medium that has:

   a a refractive index equal to that of the tissue
   b become too thick
   c been thinned too much with xylene
   d been applied to a dry slide

224 Prolonged storage of cut control slides for the stain shown below will:

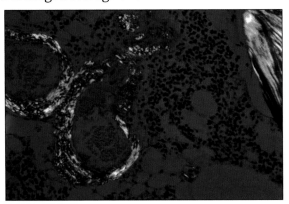

a improve polarization
b result in increased background
c cause loss of positivity
d enhance staining of old deposits

225 Filamentous structures known as "hyphae" are associated with which of the following microorganisms?

a bacteria
b protozoa
c viruses
d fungi

226 A light chain that is found in some antibodies is?

a IgA
b IgG
c IgM
d lambda

227 Tissue composed of a network of bony trabeculae separated by interconnecting bone marrow spaces is characteristic of:

a cortical bone
b woven bone
c compact bone
d cancellous bone

228 The tissue shown below is:

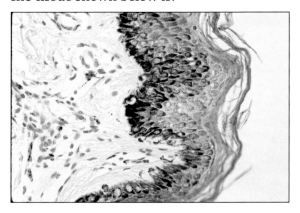

   a spleen
   b skin
   c cervix
   d esophagus

229 Which of the following is the oxidizer in the Snook and Laidlaw methods for demonstrating reticulin fibers?

   a periodic acid
   b phosphomolybdic acid
   c ferric ammonium sulfate
   d potassium permanganate

230 The second differentiating solution used in the Weil method contains sodium borate and:

   a potassium ferrocyanide
   b potassium ferricyanide
   c ferric chloride
   d ferrous sulfate

231 The property of "acid-fastness" appears to be related to the walls of organisms that contain:

   a lipid
   b protein
   c amyloid
   d iron

232 A method sometimes used for increasing the diffusion rate of dye molecules and thereby increasing the rate of staining is by increasing the dye solution:

   a temperature
   b osmolality
   c alkalinity
   d polychromasia

233 The stain shown in the image below can also be used to demonstrate:

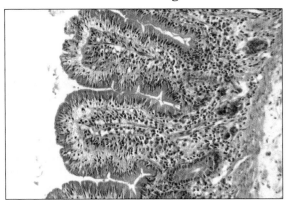

  a *Coccidioides immitis*
  b *Candida albicans*
  c *Cryptococcus neoformans*
  d *Histoplasma capsulatum*

234 Which of the following connective tissue components is sudanophilic?

  a elastin
  b reticulin
  c adipose
  d cartilage

235 Alkaline phosphatase is used in some immunohistochemical methods as the:

  a substrate
  b chromogen
  c enzyme
  d counterstain

236 A technique for demonstrating calcium wherein sections immersed in silver nitrate solution are exposed to bright light is the:

  a Schmorl
  b von Kossa
  c dopa oxidase
  d alizarin red S

237 In the Holzer method, glial fibers are stained with:

  a silver nitrate
  b crystal violet
  c orcein
  d Protargol

238 Which of the following reagents is responsible for the rose color seen in the image below?

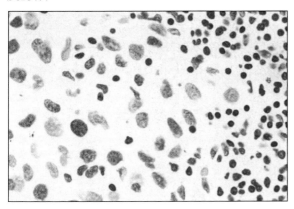

    a Schiff
    b mucicarmine
    c Congo red
    d carbol-fuchsin

239 The structures that are stained red in the image below can also be demonstrated with:

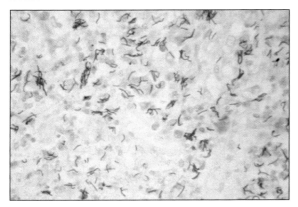

    a thioflavin T
    b acridine orange
    c periodic acid-Schiff
    d auramine-rhodamine

240 In the Masson trichrome procedure, after staining with Biebrich scarlet-acid fuchsin, sections are differentiated with:

    a 1% hydrochloric acid in 70% alcohol
    b dilute aqueous solution of acetic acid
    c phosphomolybdic-phosphotungstic acid
    d dilute ferric ammonium sulfate

241 The fibers in the image below are stained black by:

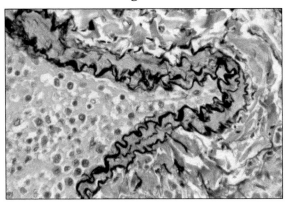

   a iron hematoxylin
   b aluminum hematoxylin
   c methenamine silver
   d diamine silver

242 Nissl substance is predominantly composed of:

   a collagenous fibers
   b neurofibrillary tangles
   c rough endoplasmic reticulum
   d microsomes and microtubules

243 In the peroxidase-antiperoxidase (PAP) method of antigen detection, the PAP complex is made in the same species as which of the following antibodies?

   a link
   b biotin-labeled
   c secondary
   d primary

ISBN 978-089189-6494   ©ASCP 2016

244 The structures stained black in the image below can also be demonstrated with which of the following stains?

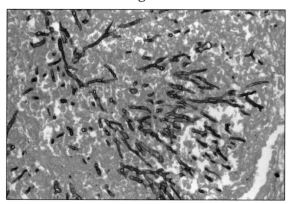

  a Gram
  b Congo red
  c Grimelius
  d periodic acid-Schiff

245 Aldehyde fuchsin to be used for elastic stains is generally stable for:

  a one week at room temperature
  b 3 to 4 weeks at 4°C
  c up to a year at 4°C
  d indefinitely

246 A combination that allows a correlative study of the cellular elements, fiber pathways, and vascular components of the nervous system is the Luxol fast blue stain combined with the:

  a PAS
  b Holmes
  c oil red O
  d PTAH

247 A possible cause of poor staining by Gomori aldehyde fuchsin solution is that:

  a fresh paraldehyde was used
  b the dye was not the correct color index
  c hydrochloric acid was used
  d 70% ethanol was used as the dye solvent

248 Argentaffin procedures will stain all of the following EXCEPT:

  a melanin
  b formalin pigment
  c enterochromaffin cells
  d calcium

249 The end-product of the reaction demonstrated in the image below is:

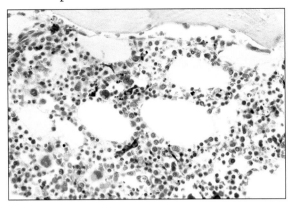

   a ferric ferrocyanide
   b ferrous ferricyanide
   c potassium ferricyanide
   d potassium ferrocyanide

250 Some dye solutions are made colorless by reduction, used for identification of specific tissue components, and then reoxidized to restore the color. The term applied to these colorless compounds is:

   a xanthanes
   b chromophoric
   c leuco
   d peroxidases

251 In neurons, chromatolysis refers to the loss of:

   a axons
   b Nissl substance
   c dendrites
   d myelin

252 Because melanin can bind and reduce silver without the use of a separate reducing agent, it is said to be:

   a argentaffin
   b amphoteric
   c argyrophilic
   d achromatic

253 In silver impregnation methods, gold chloride is used as a/an:

   a sensitizer
   b reducer
   c toner
   d oxidizer

254 The silvery-white material in the upper right corner in the image below is:

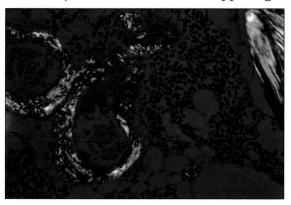

   a calcium
   b amyloid
   c muscle
   d collagen

255 A staining method for distinguishing muscle, elastic fibers, collagen, fibrin, and mucin is the:

   a Movat pentachrome
   b Gomori trichrome
   c Verhoeff-van Gieson
   d Mallory PTAH

256 The technique shown in the image below may be used for the demonstration of:

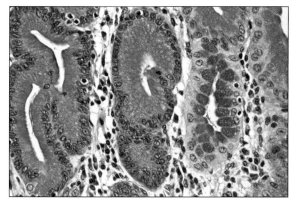

   a reducing substances
   b Nissl substance
   c glycogen
   d acid mucosubstances

257 The cells responsible for the production of the connective tissue fibers are:

    a plasma cells
    b mast cells
    c adipocytes
    d fibroblasts

258 The cells containing the black stained material in the image below are found in the:

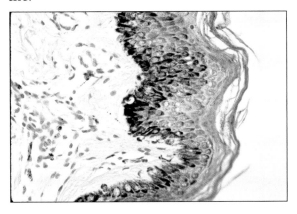

    a epidermis
    b dermis
    c hypodermis
    d deratin

259 In acid-fast staining, drying of the section after carbol-fuchsin staining should be avoided because repeated attempts at removing the insoluble compound formed by drying may result in:

    a complete decolorization of organisms
    b an opaque background
    c "beaded" red organisms
    d poor counterstaining

260 The process by which the mineral content of tissues can be studied following removal of organic tissue components is called:

    a microincineration
    b enzyme histochemistry
    c in situ hybridization
    d autoradiography

261 Insoluble compounds that resist decolorization with ether-acetone are noted on microscopic evaluation of a control section stained with the Brown-Hopps stain. The presence of these compounds is probably due to:

    a inadequate fixation
    b inadequate dehydration
    c omission of mordant during staining
    d sections being allowed to dry during staining

262 In staining methods for demonstrating reticulin, potassium permanganate, phosphomolybdic acid, and periodic acid function as:

    a reducers
    b oxidizers
    c sensitizers
    d toners

263 In the image below, myelin is demonstrated by which of the following techniques?

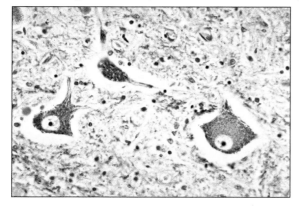

    a Weil
    b Bodian
    c Luxol fast blue
    d cresyl echt violet

264 A phosphotungstic acid-hematoxylin solution can be ripened for immediate use by adding:

    a potassium permanganate
    b aluminum sulfate
    c acetic acid
    d alcohol

265 The staining of simple fats with lipid-soluble dyes depends on:

    a Van der Waals forces
    b physical processes
    c hydrogen bonds
    d Brownian motion

266 2 eosinophilic tissue components that may be difficult to distinguish morphologically are:

    a elastic and skeletal muscle
    b cartilage and ground substance
    c collagen and smooth muscle
    d peripheral nerve and cardiac muscle

267 Small amounts of ferric iron are normally found in the:

    a liver
    b lung
    c spleen
    d kidney

268 The black stained structures in the image below are most likely stained with which of the following procedures?

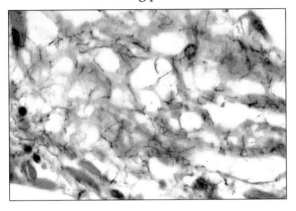

    a Truant
    b Steiner
    c Grocott
    d Gram

269 Sections are stained with Harris hematoxylin for 5 minutes and then treated with dilute hydrochloric acid. This type of staining is referred to as:

    a impregnation
    b progressive
    c regressive
    d absorption

270 The color range seen in Romanowsky stains is the result of:

    a methyl green and orange G
    b the use of pure methylene blue
    c a combination of pthalocyanine and nitro dyes
    d the combination of derivatives of methylene blue with eosin

271 The major disadvantage of using the crystal violet technique for the demonstration of amyloid is that:

   a only alpha amyloid can be demonstrated
   b it requires a polarizing microscope for verification
   c amyloid does not contrast with connective tissue
   d the preparation is not permanent

272 In the Masson trichrome stain below, the absence of some red stained tissue elements indicates:

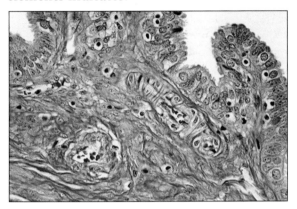

   a excellent staining quality
   b a depleted staining solution
   c an underdifferentiated stain
   d the absence of blood vessels

273 A tissue has been fixed in neutral-buffered formalin. To achieve optimum results with the Mallory PTAH stain, the microscopic sections should be:

   a cut at 10 micrometers
   b stained with freshly prepared solution
   c washed well after staining
   d mordanted in either Zenker or Bouin solution

274 When checking a control slide stained with Luxol fast blue, a good stain should show a sharp differentiation between:

   a astrocytes and microglia
   b Nissl substance and nuclei
   c gray and white matter
   d glial fibers and axons

275 Another stain that can be used to demonstrate the component stained green in the image below is:

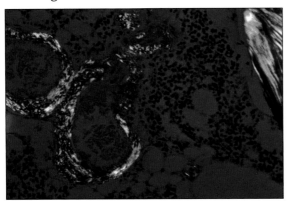

    a auramine-rhodamine
    b aldehyde fuchsin
    c thioflavin T
    d mucicarmine

276 A PTAH staining solution produces the BEST results when it is:

    a prepared fresh
    b heated to 38°C for staining
    c oxidized with ferric chloride
    d allowed to oxidize naturally

277 *Mycobacterium tuberculosis* may be demonstrated with which of the following stains?

    a crystal violet
    b leucofuchsin
    c acid fuchsin
    d carbol-fuchsin

278 Which of the following is a hydrophobic mounting medium?

    a synthetic resin
    b gelatin
    c glycerol
    d gum syrup

279 The technique shown below is used to demonstrate:

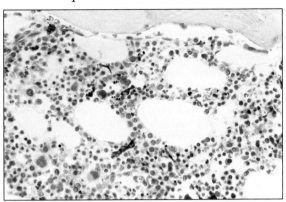

  a reducing substances
  b hemosiderin
  c hemoglobin
  d ferrous ions

280 Spirochetes in fixed tissue are BEST demonstrated by:

  a enzyme histochemistry
  b vital staining
  c metallic impregnation
  d physical methods

281 Sections stained with oil-soluble dyes must be mounted in a medium which:

  a is dissolved in a hydrocarbon
  b has a high refractive index
  c will retain lipids
  d is permanent

282 Fite, Ziehl-Neelsen, and Kinyoun are names associated with:

  a microfilaments
  b microorganisms
  c microvilli
  d microtubules

283 In the Feulgen reaction, hydrochloric acid reacts with DNA to create:

  a polynucleotides
  b base pairs
  c methyl groups
  d aldehyde groups

284 Tissue from which of the following organs should be selected as a control for the alcian blue technique, pH 2.5?

    a skin
    b kidney
    c muscle
    d colon

285 The technique shown below also may be used to demonstrate:

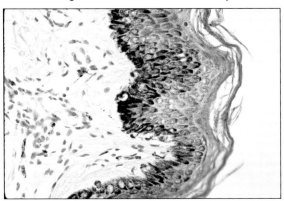

    a spirochete organisms
    b calcium deposits
    c elastic fibers
    d argentaffin cells

286 Sections were stained using the microwave oven. The tissue at the top of the slide stained darker than that at the bottom portion. To prevent this from happening in the future:

    a increase oven wattage and be sure to maintain exposure times
    b increase exposure times and be sure to maintain wattage
    c place the slides toward the back of the oven
    d remove slides from the oven and agitate solution

287 The purpose of diastase in a PAS stain is to:

    a remove glycogen from cells
    b enhance the intensity of the PAS stain
    c eliminate interfering lipoprotein
    d combine with disaccharide sugars

288 One of the components demonstrated in a section stained with Luxol fast blue and counterstained with cresyl echt violet is/are:

    a melanin granules
    b glial fibers
    c Nissl substance
    d basement membranes

289 An alcian blue stain at pH 2.5 has been requested, but no alcian blue is available. Which of the following procedures could be performed to give equivalent results?

    a Luxol fast blue
    b periodic acid-Schiff
    c colloidal iron
    d mucicarmine

290 The technique shown below is the:

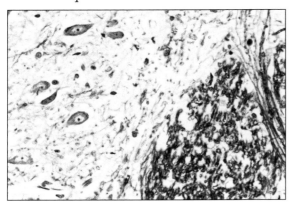

    a Bodian
    b Luxol fast blue
    c Prussian blue
    d Bielschowsky

291 In the Weil stain, borax ferricyanide differentiates the stain by:

    a changing the pH
    b bluing the hematoxylin
    c oxidation
    d excess mordant action

292 Regressive hematoxylin staining is defined as:

    a first overstaining, then differentiating
    b staining to a desired intensity, but performing no differentiation
    c applying the hematoxylin following the counterstain
    d treating the sections with a mordant and then hematoxylin

293 Which of the following may be used to stain glycogen, polysaccharides, and glycoproteins?

    a peroxidase
    b Sudan black B
    c periodic acid-Schiff (PAS)
    d nitroblue tetrazolium (NBT)

294 Poor results may be obtained in the stain shown below if the:

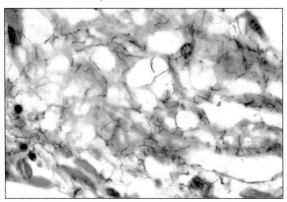

   a tissue was fixed in neutral buffered formalin
   b reducing solution contained hydroquinone
   c glassware used was not chemically cleaned
   d sections are heated in any step

295 A fresh solution of equal parts of potassium ferrocyanide and hydrochloric acid
     gives a positive reaction with:

   a iron
   b hemofuscin
   c ceroid
   d argentaffin granules

296 Bouin-fixed tissue is unsatisfactory for:

   a acid-fast stains
   b the Feulgen reaction
   c argentaffin reactions
   d mast cell demonstration

297 Which of the following procedures should be selected for the demonstration of
     axons?

   a Luxol fast blue
   b Bodian
   c cresyl echt violet
   d Holzer

298 A mordant in combination with a dye:

   a functions as a neutralizer
   b decolorizes on dehydration
   c acts as a differentiator
   d forms a dye lake

299 Delafield hematoxylin is most commonly aged with:

  a alcohol
  b light
  c heat
  d vacuum

300 The technique shown below is used for the demonstration of:

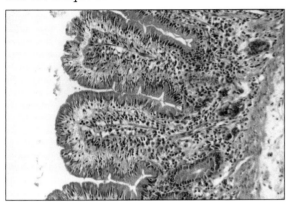

  a acid mucosubstances
  b neutral mucosubstances
  c starch granules
  d glycogen

301 Generally, acid dyes are differentiated in solutions that are weakly:

  a acidic
  b basic
  c neutral
  d amphoteric

302 An amphoteric substance is one that can act as a/an:

  a acid
  b base
  c salt
  d acid or base

303 The substance stained rose-red in the image below is:

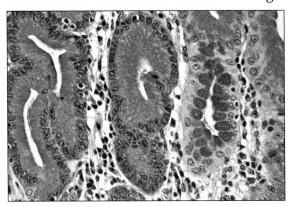

    a glycogen

    b an acid mucosubstance

    c a neutral mucosubstance

    d carboxylated mucosubstance

304 Microscopic sections stained with H&E show a lack of nuclear staining even though the hematoxylin is well ripened and all other solutions are fresh. Which of the following factors could explain the poor results?

    a the slides were left too long in the neutralizer

    b prolonged storage of wet tissue in unbuffered formalin

    c the pH of the hematoxylin is between 2 and 2.4

    d the embedding paraffin is too hot

305 Microscopic review of H&E stained sections reveals that the eosin is very pale. This is most likely due to:

    a inadequate rinsing after neutralization

    b incomplete dehydration after eosin

    c the use of acetified eosin

    d improper clearing

306 The staining mechanism whereby dye adheres to the surface of structures is called:

    a absorption

    b impregnation

    c adsorption

    d orthochromasia

307 Weigert hematoxylin solution is generally unsatisfactory for use after 3 to 4:

    a hours

    b days

    c weeks

    d months

308 Which of the structures listed should be red in the poor Masson trichrome stain
     seen below?

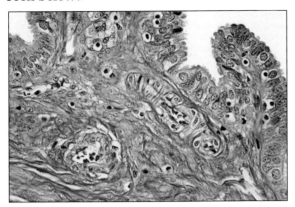

a nuclei
b collagen
c epithelium
d reticulin

309 In a routine staining series, slides placed in xylene for clearing prior to
     coverslipping have an opaque appearance. This is most likely due to incomplete:

a neutralization
b dehydration
c deparaffinization
d differentiation

310 Tissue sections were stained for the recommended time with an H&E procedure
     using Harris hematoxylin. A quality control check shows pale nuclear staining. A
     likely cause of this could be:

a too much alum mordant in the stock hematoxylin solution
b excessive treatment with the bluing agent
c too much time in the differentiating solution
d prolonged dehydration and clearing

311 Dyes used for nuclear staining are:

a acid
b basic
c neutral
d amphoteric

312 A stock solution of Harris hematoxylin is being prepared for use in the routine H&E procedure. To make it an effective nuclear stain, the dye must be:

a amphoteric
b negatively charged
c oxidized
d fresh

313 The stain seen in the image below is:

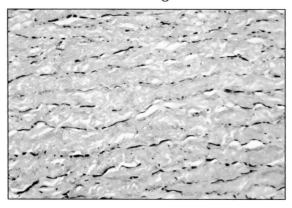

a satisfactory
b underdifferentiated
c overdifferentiated
d poorly counterstained

314 An antigenic determinant present on a complete antigenic molecule is known as a/an:

a antibody class
b immunogen
c immunoglobulin
d epitope

315 A dye that absorbs light and then emits its own light at a longer wavelength is known as:

a conjugated
b a fluorochrome
c a chromogen
d polarization

The following items (*) have been identified as more appropriate for entry level histotechnologists.

*316 A fungus that can be demonstrated with various stains for acidic mucins is:

    a *Candida albicans*
    b *Histoplasma capsulatum*
    c *Cryptococcus neoformans*
    d *Coccidioides immitis*

*317 ATPase stains are done on a muscle biopsy at pH 9.4, 4.6, and 4.3. The slides for pH 9.4 and pH 4.3 show good differentiation of the type I and type II fibers, and although the slide done at pH 4.6 shows differentiation of the type I and type II fibers, it does not show differentiation of the type IIA and IIB fibers. This indicates that the:

    a ammonium sulfide solution is old
    b the pH should be modified on the 4.6 stain
    c calcium should be omitted from the incubating solution
    d the results of the pH 4.6 stain duplicate those of the pH 4.3 and could be omitted

*318 A pathologic condition characterized by abnormal deposits of iron in the liver is called:

    a hemachrosis
    b hemochromatosis
    c hemadostenosis
    d hematotoxicosis

*319 A student has turned in the alcian blue stain seen below for her final exam. The student had to select the block, cut and stain the section. The supervisor should tell the student that the slide is unacceptable because:

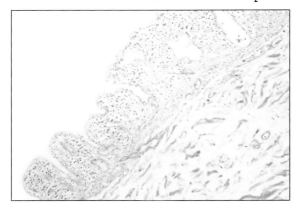

    a small intestine is not a good tissue to demonstrate the alcian blue stain
    b the connective tissue has picked up the alcian blue
    c no epithelium is present to demonstrate acidic mucins
    d nuclear fast red should not have been chosen as the counterstain

*320 An enzyme technique that will demonstrate denervated muscle fibers and motor end plates is the:

   a NAD-diaphorase
   b acid phosphatase
   c phosphorylase
   d alpha-naphthyl acetate esterase

*321 Which of the following procedures will demonstrate *Helicobacter pylori* most rapidly in a laboratory without a microwave oven?

   a Steiner and Steiner
   b Diff-Quik
   c Truant
   d Dieterle

*322 A research project requires the demonstration of lysosomes on frozen sections of muscle tissue. The BEST procedure would be:

   a ATPase, pH 4.2
   b phosphorylase
   c acid phosphatase
   d succinic dehydrogenase

*323 In the PAS reaction, development of the final colored product is achieved by:

   a oxidation of aldehyde groups
   b extraction of diastase-sensitive structures
   c restoration of the quinoid structure
   d cleavage of 1:2 glycol groups

*324 Mucicarmine positive material is noted in the cytoplasm of poorly differentiated malignant cells. This finding is indicative of a/an:

   a adenocarcinoma
   b squamous carcinoma
   c leiomyosarcoma
   d large cell lymphoma

*325 One of the rare enzyme techniques that can be performed on paraffin sections is the:

   a naphthol AS-D chloroacetate esterase
   b succinic dehydrogenase
   c alkaline phosphatase
   d ATPase, pH 9.4

*326 The activity of succinic dehydrogenase will be destroyed:

    a at 37°C
    b at pH 7.6
    c by freezing
    d by fixation

*327 The final reaction product in the technique shown below is:

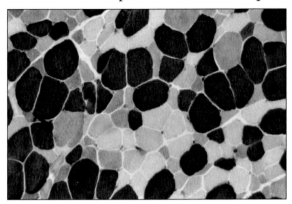

    a calcium phosphate
    b cobalt phosphate
    c calcium sulfide
    d cobalt sulfide

*328 Acid phosphatase falls under the basic enzyme-reaction classification of:

    a oxidoreductases
    b transferases
    c hydrolases
    d isomerases

*329 Structures that speed up the rate of enzyme reactions are known as:

    a cofactors
    b coenzymes
    c substrates
    d phosphatases

*330 Enzymes that catalyze chemical reactions in biologic systems are:

    a metals
    b carbohydrates
    c proteins
    d substrates

*331 A procedure that demonstrates some carcinoid tumors as well as alpha cells of the pancreas is the:

    a Fontana-Masson
    b Warthin-Starry
    c Grimelius
    d periodic acid-Schiff

*332 A patient is suspected of having McArdle disease, which is a glycogen storage disease affecting skeletal muscle. This disease is BEST demonstrated with which of the following techniques?

    a alpha-naphthyl acetate esterase
    b ATPase, pH 9.4 and 4.3
    c acid phosphatase
    d phosphorylase

*333 The organism stained black in the image seen below is most likely:

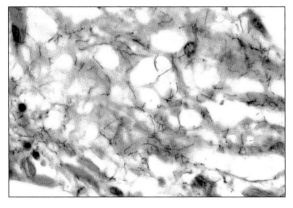

    a *Helicobacter pylori*
    b *Treponema pallidum*
    c *Mycobacterium leprae*
    d *Psuedomonas aeruginosa*

*334 Experiments have shown that a particular lipid fraction known as mycolic acid exists within the cell walls of:

    a *Mycobacterium tuberculosis*
    b *Pneumocystis jirovecii*
    c *Actinomyces bovis*
    d *Candida albicans*

*335 Antibody molecules can belong to one of 5 immunoglobulin classes. The antibody class most frequently used in immunohistochemistry is:

a IgM
b IgE
c IgG
d IgA

*336 The red-brown nuclear staining sometimes seen with hematoxylin is generally caused by:

a evaporation of the solution
b too much treatment with alkaline solutions
c the solution breaking down
d excess ammonium aluminum sulfate

*337 In immunohistochemical procedures, excess background staining can be reduced by:

a using whole serum antibodies
b applying a more concentrated antibody solution
c incubating for a shorter time in the primary antibody
d pretreating with nonimmune serum from the same animal species as the secondary antibody

*338 The brown stained structure in the image below is the:

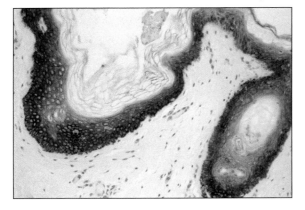

a epithelium
b dermis
c lamina propria
d adventia

*339 Compounds and tissue elements that fluoresce naturally without the use of fluorochrome dyes are said to have the property of:

    a autofluorescence
    b secondary fluorescence
    c autoradiographic properties
    d dichroism

*340 Which of the following fungi may appear as a mixture of budding yeast cells and pseudohypha elements in infected tissue?

    a *Aspergillus fumigatus*
    b *Candida albicans*
    c *Histoplasma capsulatum*
    d *Cryptococcus neoformans*

*341 Mycotic diseases that go beyond superficial or cutaneous involvement to affect vital organs and cause extensive disease and even death are referred to as:

    a subcutaneous
    b systemic
    c dermatosis
    d calcific

*342 The specific area of the central nervous system seen below is the:

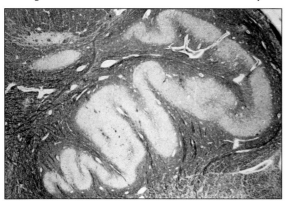

    a cerebellum
    b cerebral cortex
    c pons
    d medulla

*343 In a suspected case of Alzheimer disease, a staining method that may help confirm the diagnosis is:

    a oil red O
    b H&E
    c Bielschowsky
    d Luxol fast blue

*344 Type I muscle fibers demonstrate more positive staining results than type II fibers in a dehydrogenase enzyme procedure such as:

   a NADH diaphorase
   b PASH
   c DOPA oxidase
   d phosphorylase

*345 An orthochromatic dye stains tissue:

   a different from the color of the dye itself
   b not at all
   c only partially
   d the color of the dye itself

*346 A possible cause of the problem seen below is:

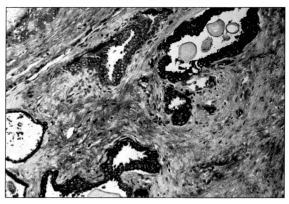

   a reagents used in the wrong order
   b primary antibody too concentrated
   c reagents are expired
   d epitope enhancement method incorrectly done

*347 Which of the following methods should be used for the demonstration of rickettsias?

   a Grocott
   b Giemsa
   c Gridley
   d Fite

*348 The succinic dehydrogenase technique will stain only:

   a sarcoplasmic reticulin
   b Z-band material
   c mitochondria
   d motor endplates

*349 A good control for the antibody Cam 5.2 is a:

    a lymphoma
    b carcinoma
    c melanoma
    d sarcoma

*350 A rhabdomyosarcoma is suspected in a biopsy submitted to the laboratory. To aid in making a definitive diagnosis, a helpful nonimmunologic stain would be the:

    a phosphotungstic acid-hematoxylin (PTAH)
    b Gomori aldehyde fuchsin
    c Mayer mucicarmine
    d Verhoeff-van Gieson

*351 The technique shown below is often used in the diagnosis of:

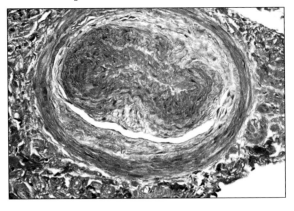

    a pancreatic islet cell disease
    b mycotic diseases
    c blood vessel invasion by tumor
    d cirrhosis of the liver

*352 In lung tissue, coated asbestos fibers can be made more visible by staining with:

    a Schiff reagent
    b silver nitrate
    c Prussian blue reaction
    d aldehyde fuchsin

*353 Which of the following cells is responsible for immunoglobulin production?

    a histiocyte
    b mast
    c neutrophil
    d plasma

*354 Melanosis coli is a condition characterized by abnormal deposits of pigment that will give a positive reaction in which of the following procedures?

a Congo red
b Grimelius
c Schmorl
d von Kossa

*355 The primary problem seen in Luxol fast blue-cresyl echt violet stain seen below could most likely be corrected by:

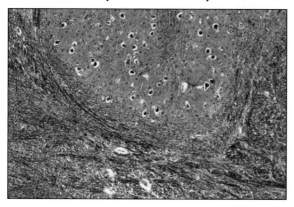

a verifying the addition of acid to the cresyl echt violet
b decreasing the temperature of the cresyl echt violet stain
c checking the preparation of the Luxol fast blue solution
d increasing the time of the Luxol fast blue differentiation

*356 Astrocytes can be demonstrated by using the antibody that is specific for:

a vimentin
b S-100
c cytokeratin
d GFAP

*357 The combining sites of an antibody molecule are the:

a constant region
b hinge regions
c variable regions
d Fc fragments

*358 Melanins are bleached by all of the following EXCEPT:

a hydrogen peroxide
b chromic acid
c potassium permanganate
d acetone

*359 The enzyme technique shown below utilizes:

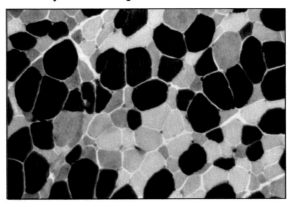

   a self-colored substrate
   b metallic impregnation
   c metallic precipitation
   d molecular rearrangement

*360 Of the following, the BEST stain to demonstrate loss of muscle striations caused by dystrophic change is the:

   a Masson trichrome
   b Verhoeff-van Gieson
   c Mallory PTAH
   d Gomori trichrome

*361 The tissue shown is a good control for which of the antibodies listed?

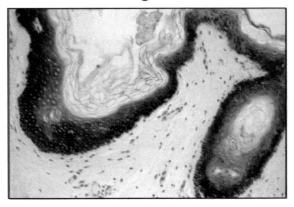

   a AE1/AE3
   b CD20
   c CD3
   d LCA

*362 The amorphous transparent gel-like material that forms the bulk of extracellular content in connective tissue is known as:

 a basal lamina
 b lamina propria
 c mesenchyme
 d ground substance

*363 Small eosinophilic inclusions found in the cytoplasm of neurons in patients infected with the rabies virus are called:

 a Barr bodies
 b Negri bodies
 c Russell bodies
 d Donovan bodies

*364 When selecting reagents for peroxidase-anti-peroxidase (PAP) staining, the PAP complex should be prepared in the same (or a closely related) animal species as the:

 a antigen of study
 b secondary antibody
 c primary antibody
 d bridging antibody

*365 Tumors derived from argentaffin cells of the gastrointestinal tract fall in the general classification of:

 a adenomas
 b apudomas
 c carcinomas
 d sarcomas

*366 A fungal disease characterized by narrow-based budding and carminophilia of yeast organisms is:

 a blastomycosis
 b cryptococcosis
 c histoplasmosis
 d candidiasis

*367 A "Maltese cross" configuration is produced in tissue sections by polarization of:

 a calcium oxalate
 b uric acid
 c talcum powder
 d lipofuscin

*368 A pigment occurring in *Plasmodium* parasites that is closely related to formalin pigment is:

  a hemoglobin
  b melanin
  c malarial
  d lipofuscin

*369 In immunohistochemical reactions using horseradish peroxidase, a solution of hydrogen peroxide in methanol is used to:

  a block endogenous peroxidase
  b enhance background staining
  c affect reactivity of antibodies and antigens
  d intensify the coloring products

*370 Luxol fast blue dye has a structural formula closely related to that of:

  a methylene blue
  b sky blue
  c Nile blue sulfate
  d alcian blue 8GX

*371 The stain shown in the image below is most likely the:

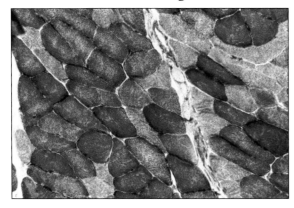

  a NADH diaphorase
  b acid phosphatase
  c phosphorylase
  d ATPase

*372 In immunohistochemical staining of formalin fixed tissue, heat-induced epitope retrieval:

  a increases background staining
  b enhances primary staining
  c is needed to demonstrate all tissue antigens
  d has precise endpoints

*373 The tissue shown in the image below has been stained with the Masson trichrome. After reviewing the slide, the technologists should:

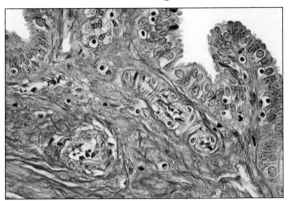

  a repeat the stain using heat
  b label the slide and send it out
  c decolorize and restain the slide
  d repeat, ensuring mordanting in Bouin solution

*374 Following immunohistochemical staining, both the positive control and the specimen show weak staining. The most likely cause is that:

  a both tissues contain free antigen
  b epitope retrieval was incorrectly done
  c staining steps were performed in the wrong order
  d the hydrogen peroxide blocking step was omitted

*375 A protozoan that causes outbreaks of severe and relentless diarrhea among patients with acquired immunodeficiency syndrome (AIDS) is:

  a *Cryptosporidium muris*
  b *Leishmania donovani*
  c *Giardia lamblia*
  d *Toxoplasma gondii*

*376 The problem seen below is occurring on numerous slides. It is most likely caused by:

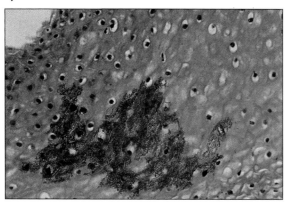

    a retracted mounting medium
    b mounting medium on top of cover glass
    c slide drying before mounting
    d incomplete dehydration of the slides

*377 Immunoperoxidase stained tissues show a reaction of red blood cells and granulocytes with the chromogenic substrate. The most likely cause of this reaction is that:

    a the tissues contain antigen that reacted with the primary antiserum
    b the specimens were improperly counterstained
    c endogenous peroxidase was not blocked
    d the specimens were allowed to dry during the staining procedure

*378 "Mycoses" is the term used to describe diseases caused by:

    a bacteria
    b viruses
    c fungi
    d protozoa

*379 Myelin contains protein, cholesterol, cerebrosides, and:

    a fatty acids
    b phospholipids
    c mucoproteins
    d endoplasmic reticulum

*380 In the procedure seen below, the splitting of purines and pyrimidines from the sugar-phosphate groupings of DNA is called:

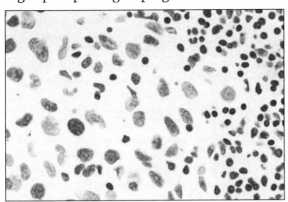

   a autolysis
   b synthesis
   c hydrolysis
   d extraction

*381 *Alipia felis* (cat-scratch disease) bacteria can be demonstrated with the:

   a microwave modification of Warthin-Starry
   b Fontana-Masson silver impregnation
   c Ziehl-Neelson carbol fuchsin
   d Grocott methenamine silver

*382 Rickettsiae are related to which of the following classifications of microorganisms?

   a molds
   b yeasts
   c bacteria
   d protozoa

*383 Which of the following procedures is most suitable for demonstrating secretory granules in a carcinoid tumor?

   a Wilder reticulin
   b PAS-aniline blue
   c Snook
   d Grimelius

*384 Cell blocks prepared on cytology specimens:

   a provide little additional diagnostic information
   b require a special method of dehydration and clearing
   c are very difficult to prepare
   d make it easier to do special stains

*385 The primary cells involved in immune responses belong to the lymphoreticular system and are found in large numbers in which of the following sites in the body?

    a heart, lungs, liver, brain
    b skeletal muscle, liver, pancreas, skin
    c thymus, lymph nodes, spleen, bone marrow
    d kidney, liver, adrenal, heart

*386 The enzyme involved in the technique shown below belongs to which of the following classes?

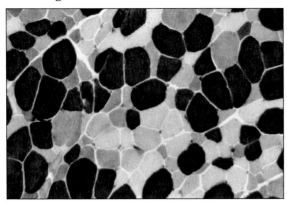

    a lipases
    b hydrolases
    c transferases
    d oxidoreductases

*387 Fixation in a primary chromate fixative is essential if chromaffin substance is to be demonstrated by which of the following procedures?

    a modified Steiner
    b Gomori iron
    c trichrome-new fuchsin
    d Schmorl

*388 Chromaffin-cell tumors of the adrenal gland are known as:

    a adenomas
    b carcinoids
    c leiomyosarcoma
    d pheochromocytomas

*389 A Papanicolaou stained smear shows only blue-green cytoplasm in all cells. No pink cytoplasm is noted. The cytology preparatory technician should be cautioned about:

    a fixing too long in 95% alcohol
    b decreasing the time in the EA solution
    c over-rinsing the slides
    d acidifying the OG-6

*390 ATPase stains were performed at pH 9.4 and 4.3. Each of these stains shows large type grouping of both dark and light staining fibers. The patterns of dark and light stained fibers are reversed at the different pHs. This result is most likely due to:

    a prolonged incubation
    b a myopathic disease process
    c depleted staining reagents
    d a neuropathic disease process

*391 The final reaction product in the technique shown below is:

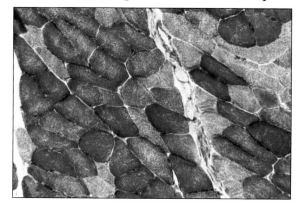

    a cobalt sulfide
    b azo dye
    c formazan
    d amylose

*392 Controls for immunohistochemistry can be divided into 3 major categories. All of the follow are control categories EXCEPT:

    a absorption
    b positive
    c antigen
    d negative

*393 The technique shown below depends on the use of:

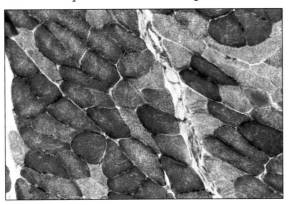

  a 4 to 5 μm sections
  b frozen sections of unfixed tissue
  c fixation following frozen sectioning
  d antigen retrieval solutions

*394 In addition to the heat employed, an important factor in heat-induced epitope retrieval is the:

  a enzyme solution selected
  b use of a metallic co-factor
  c composition of the retrieval solution
  d solution have a pH of 10.0 or higher

*395 The laboratory has received the report from the Histology Quality Improvement Program concerning the last slides submitted for evaluation. The H&E stains were downgraded because only 2 shades of eosin could be seen. To get the recommended 3 shades of eosin, the H&E procedure should be changed by:

  a decreasing the staining time in eosin
  b increasing the water rinse following bluing
  c raising the pH of the eosin solution to above 7.0
  d increasing the time in the lower dilution of dehydrating alcohols

*396 When staining renal biopsy sections for examination by fluorescence microscopy:

  a tissue antigens are "stained" by fluorochrome labeled antibody
  b tissue antibodies are "stained" by fluorochrome labeled antigens
  c fluorescent dyes are sandwiched between antigen and antibody
  d fluorescent dyes are bound to tissue with heavy metal mordants

*397 In paraffin sections, hepatitis B surface antigen may be demonstrated with:

  a Congo red
  b alcian blue
  c orcein
  d Bielschowsky

*398 Which of the following cells are found predominantly in the central nervous system?

   a Schwann
   b Golgi
   c ganglion
   d astrocytes

*399 After microscopic review of the control slide shown below, the technician responsible should be:

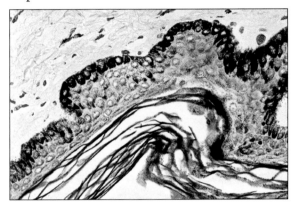

   a asked to shorten future impregnation times
   b complemented on a stain well done
   c questioned on the reducing solution used
   d reminded to use the melanin bleach

*400 The point of contact between an axon of one neuron and the dendrite of another neuron is called a(n):

   a link
   b synapse
   c attachment
   d contact

*401 *Listeria monocytogenes*, the cause of a rare form of meningitis, can BEST be demonstrated in a paraffin section with which of the following staining procedures?

   a hematoxylin and eosin
   b Ziehl-Neelsen
   c Grocott
   d Gram

*402 The problem seen in the Masson trichrome stain shown below was most likely the result of:

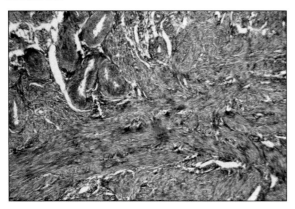

   a improper drying of the section
   b incomplete deparaffinization
   c pathologically altered collagen
   d using old or depleted reagents

*403 The use of heat and prolonged staining with Ziehl-Neelsen carbol fuchsin may be used to demonstrate the acid-fast characteristics of certain:

   a proteins
   b mucins
   c spermatozoa
   d lipofuscins

*404 Immunologic staining can BEST be adapted for localization of surface antigens by electron microscopy following staining with:

   a amino-ethylcarbazole
   b colloidal gold
   c diaminobenzidine
   d silver nitrate

*405 A tumor that is positive with the LCA antibody is known as a:

   a neuroblastoma
   b lymphoma
   c carcinoma
   d sarcoma

*406 The chromogen used in the image below was most likely:

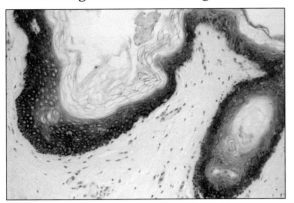

   a AEC
   b PAP
   c DAB
   d FITC

*407 Organisms found on gastric mucosa that are the presumptive cause of gastritis, have a curved configuration, and may be stained with silver impregnation procedures are most likely:

   a *Borrelia burgdorferi*
   b *Treponema pallidum*
   c *Leptospira interrogans*
   d *Helicobacter pylori*

*408 The viability of the primary staining solution used in the procedure illustrated below can be checked with:

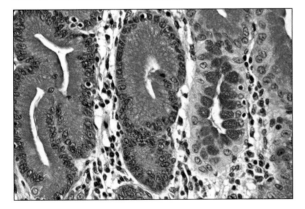

   a acetic acid
   b a pH meter
   c formaldehyde
   d sodium bisulfite

*409 A good procedure for determining cellularity during procedures, such as fine-needle aspiration is a/an:

    a toluidine blue wet film
    b rapid hematoxylin and eosin
    c Wright stain
    d aldehyde fuchsin

*410 A liver biopsy from a patient with suspected Wilson disease shows cirrhosis. This diagnosis could be confirmed by using a rubeanic acid stain to demonstrate the presence of:

    a bile
    b copper
    c lipofuscin
    d hematoidin

*411 The periodic acid-Schiff (PAS) procedure will stain *Coccidioides immitis* because the organisms:

    a are argyrophilic
    b exhibit metachromasia
    c contain carbohydrates
    d reduce Schiff reagent

*412 In immunohistochemical staining, a limitation of polyclonal antibody techniques as opposed to monoclonal antibody techniques is the:

    a greater cross-reactivity with similar antigens
    b more difficult production of polyclonal antibodies
    c limited availability of antisera
    d extreme specificity of polyclonals

*413 The stain illustrated in the image below is a Luxol fast blue-cresyl echt violet stain. For this stain, cresyl echt violet should stain ONLY the:

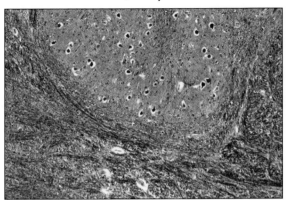

    a glial cells
    b myelin sheath
    c nuclei and Nissl substance
    d neurofibrillary tangles

*414 Sarcomas are negative with all of the antibodies listed below EXCEPT:

    a HMB-45
    b GFAP
    c vimentin
    d cytokeratin

*415 One of the most widespread and prevalent of the mycotic diseases in man is:

    a coccidioidomycosis
    b protothecosis
    c candidiasis
    d rhinosporidiosis

*416 The stain shown below was done at pH 4.6. The very dark fibers are type:

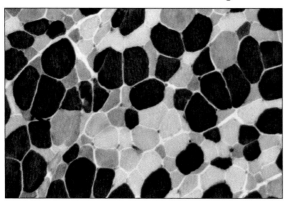

  a I
  b IIA
  c IIB
  d IIC

*417 In addition to being associated with a wide variety of neurons, nervous tissue is also closely associated with non-neuronal cells, including:

  a keratinocytes and melanocytes
  b Langerhans and Merkel cells
  c histiocytes and mesangial cells
  d Schwann and glial cells

*418 Microscopic review of H&E stained sections of liver shows some blue staining of the cytoplasm. This is most likely caused by:

  a a marked amount of rough endoplasmic reticulum
  b overstaining with Mayer hematoxylin
  c inadequate differentiation of the hematoxylin
  d too much time in the bluing solution

*419 The primary function of auxochromes in artificial dyes is to:

  a deepen the color
  b change the dye shade
  c give the dye affinity for the tissue
  d stabilize the dye compound when in solution

*420 When a slide like this is submitted for evaluation by the Histology Quality Improvement Program, one of the evaluator's comments that should be expected is:

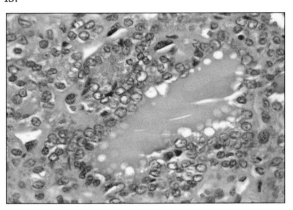

   a nuclear stain too dark
   b incomplete fixation
   c eosin staining too light
   d only one shade of eosin noted

*421 Chromaffin cells of the adrenal gland are located in the:

   a zona glomerulosa
   b zona reticularis
   c zona fasciculata
   d medulla

*422 The refractive index of the resinous mounting media used for stained sections should be approximately:

   a 0.52 to 0.85
   b 1.30 to 1.41
   c 1.53 to 1.54
   d 1.60 to 1.73

*423 The Bielschowsky method involves double-impregnation of brain sections with silver nitrate solution. The reducing agent used in this method is:

   a hydroquinone
   b phenol
   c sodium sulfite
   d formaldehyde

*424 All of the following microorganisms will stain with carbol-fuchsin solution EXCEPT:

   a *Treponema pallidum*
   b *Mycobacterium leprae*
   c *Nocardia asteroides*
   d *Mycobacterium tuberculosis*

*425 The most common basic auxochrome group encountered in dye chemistry is:

   a $-NH_2$
   b $-COOH$
   c $-OH$
   d $-N=N$

*426 Nissl substance can be demonstrated by staining parallel sections before and after extraction with:

   a diastase
   b ribonuclease
   c hyaluronidase
   d deoxyribonuclease

*427 A common acidic auxochrome is:

   a $-COOH$
   b $-NH_2$
   c $-N=N-$
   d $-NO_2$

*428 A rhabdomyosarcoma is a malignant neoplasm of:

   a smooth muscle
   b skeletal muscle
   c epithelium
   d glands

*429 The stain shown below:

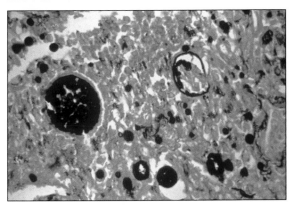

  a is an excellent Grocott stain
  b has been over impregnated
  c has not been oxidized properly
  d demonstrates *Histoplasma* organisms

*430 The enzyme classification of hydrolases includes all of the following EXCEPT:

  a esterases
  b phosphatases
  c peptidases
  d phosphorylases

*431 If the mucoid capsule of the fungus is intact, which of the following fungi can be differentially stained by Mayer mucicarmine?

  a *Histoplasma capsulatum*
  b *Coccidioides immitis*
  c *Cryptococcus neoformans*
  d *Candida albicans*

*432 Although hematoxylin solutions generally require a mordant, they may be used without a mordant to demonstrate:

  a calcium
  b copper
  c lipids
  d glycogen

*433 The phenomenon shown in the image below is known as:

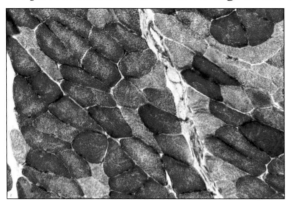

 a myopathy
 b phagocytosis
 c atrophy
 d type grouping

*434 ATPase stained sections are retrieved after storage for several years. Microscopic evaluation shows marked fading of the stain. This indicates that:

 a normal fading with time has occurred
 b the storage conditions were inappropriate
 c the pH of the solutions was not stabilized
 d the ammonium sulfide was too dilute when used

*435 Protease is used in immunohistochemistry for::

 a the enzyme label for some antibodies
 b as the chromogen for alkaline phosphatase
 c as the blocking agent for avidin
 d for enzyme-induced retrieval

*436 The method of choice for demonstrating calcium phosphate is the:

 a Pizzolato
 b von Kossa
 c Schmorl
 d rubeanic acid

*437 In the avidin-biotin complex (ABC) immunohistochemical procedure:

 a the primary antiserum is avidin-labeled
 b no conjugation steps are involved in the reaction
 c the ABC complex binds to biotin-labeled secondary antibody
 d the bridging antiserum is added in excess

ISBN 978-089189-6494 ©ASCP 2016

*438 The problem seen in the image below can be corrected in the future by:

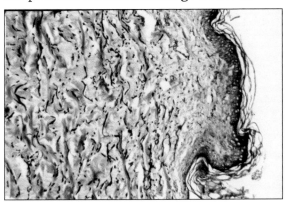

    a no corrective action is needed in this stain
    b increase the differentiation of the elastic tissue
    c ensuring that the picric acid solution is saturated
    d decrease the amount of acid fuchsin in the van Gieson

*439 When no immunostaining of either the patient or positive control tissue is seen, one explanation might be that:

    a delayed or inadequate fixation of the patient tissue
    b the patient tissue was fixed by a different method than the control
    c uneven deposition of the detection reagent
    d an incorrect primary antibody was applied

*440 One advantage of using diaminobenzidine (DAB) rather than aminoethylcarbazole (AEC) as the chromogen is:

    a a permanent preparation is obtained
    b the contrast with melanotic lesions is better
    c the clarity of the section is decreased
    d there is no intensification available

*441 Which of the following procedures can be used to demonstrate *Giardia duodenalis* (*lamblia*)?

    a Giemsa
    b Grocott
    c Brown and Brenn
    d Kinyoun

*442 The enzyme involved in the technique shown below belongs to which of the following classes?

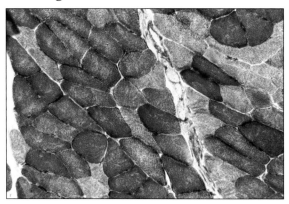

  a lipases
  b hydrolases
  c transferases
  d oxidoreductases

*443 Which of the following procedures will demonstrate *Borrelia burgdorferi*?

  a Fite
  b Gridley
  c Steiner
  d Truant

*444 An undifferentiated malignant neoplasm stains positive for leukocyte common antigen and negative for carcinoembryonic antigen and cytokeratin. Therefore, the origin of these malignant cells is most likely:

  a epithelial
  b melanocytic
  c neural
  d lymphatic

*445 A major reason for selecting a peroxidase-antiperoxidase (PAP) staining technique over direct or indirect conjugate methods is that, with PAP, there is/are:

  a fewer steps involved
  b better blockage of endogenous peroxidase
  c increased sensitivity of antigen detection
  d less hazard of exposure to potential carcinogens

*446 There is very weak alcian blue staining in structures that are expected to be positive. What is the most likely cause?

    a PAS procedure was used as the counterstain
    b alcian blue reagent is pH 2.5
    c section was fixed in 10% NB formalin
    d there was poor hydration during the deparaffinization steps

*447 A tumor that is thought to be associated with asbestos exposure is:

    a dysgerminoma
    b hepatocellular carcinoma
    c hypernephroma
    d mesothelioma

*448 Which of the following immunohistochemical techniques is mainly confined to the demonstration of immunoglobulin and complement in frozen sections of skin and renal biopsies:

    a polymer chain 2-step indirect
    b unlabeled antibody-enzyme complex
    c traditional direct technique
    d avidin-biotin

*449 The tissue shown in the technique below is:

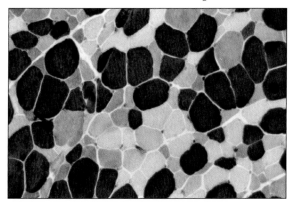

    a cardiac muscle
    b skeletal muscle
    c pancreas
    d liver

*450 All of the following are used for heat-induced antigen retrieval EXCEPT:

    a microwave oven
    b pressure cooker
    c 60° oven
    d 95-98° water bath

*451 The proteins that form the thick and thin filaments of skeletal muscle fibers are:

   a fibrin and fibrinogen
   b collagen and tropocollagen
   c actin and myosin
   d thrombin and prothrombin

*452 A birefringent reaction product is produced following staining of calcium deposits with which of the following stains?

   a Schmorl
   b von Kossa
   c dopa oxidase
   d alizarin red S

*453 The pathologists want to try using a different fixative for all tissues. Which of the following times would most likely have to be adjusted for the stain shown below?

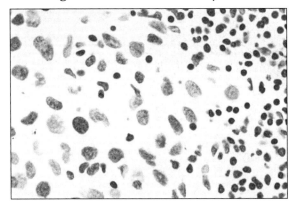

   a hydrolysis with 1 N HCL
   b staining in Schiff reagent
   c sulfurous acid rinses
   d choice of counterstain

*454 In the acid phosphatase technique, the reaction product is formed by the coupling of a diazonium salt and a/an:

   a azo group
   b naphthol group
   c thymol molecule
   d acetate salt

*455 Neuritic plaques of Alzheimer disease consist of abnormal cell processes, often in close proximity to deposits of:

   a amyloid
   b phospholipids
   c neuromelanin
   d astrocytes

ISBN 978-089189-6494 ©ASCP 2016

*456 Validation of a new antibody involves using all of the following EXCEPT:

a multiple chromogens
b multiple retrieval methods
c serial dilutions
d several appropriate file cases

*457 A trainee is having trouble counterstaining a Grocott fungal stain with light green. The counterstain just is not taking. One of the most appropriate questions would be to ask if the:

a light green was too concentrated
b section was oxidized
c light green was acidified
d gold chloride solution was 0.1%

*458 The Papanicolaou counterstained smears look dirty and not optimal. The cytopreparatory technician should be reminded to:

a shorten the time in the bluing agent
b ensure clean alcoholic rinses after counterstains
c follow counterstains with absolute alcohol only
d use EA-36 for specimen with large amount of mucus

*459 The sites of dark red staining in α-naphthyl acetate esterase stain below are:

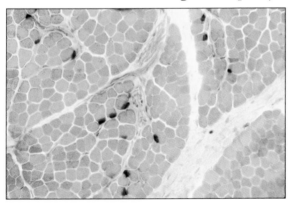

a motor end-plates
b inflammatory cells
c denervated muscle cells
d nemaline rods

*460 When the ABC complex detection system is used in immunohistochemistry, the possibility of false positive staining is high in some tissues such as:

a pancreas
b thyroid
c pineal body
d liver

*461 The diagnosis of Alzheimer disease is based on the presence of neurofibrillary tangles and neuritic plaques in the:

    a spinal cord
    b cortex
    c medulla oblongata
    d cerebellum

*462 Silver nitrate is not available to perform a requested basement membrane stain. Another method that can be used is:

    a alcian blue-aldehyde fuchsin
    b Masson trichrome
    c periodic acid-Schiff
    d Weigert resorcin fuchsin

*463 A trainee about to perform a Feulgen reaction reports that no Feulgen reagent can be found in the lab. The trainee should be told to look instead for which of the following reagents?

    a Schmorl
    b van Gieson
    c Schiff
    d Fouchet

*464 The HMB-45 antibody is associated with the demonstration of:

    a melanin
    b hemoglobin
    c hemosiderin
    d lipofuscin

*465 Microscopic evaluation of a section of brain stained with the Holzer technique should show:

    a dark blue myelin
    b blue to purple glial fibers
    c black axons and dendrites
    d violet Nissl substance

*466 Microscopic evaluation of an auramine-rhodamine stained control section shows minute, shiny, orange structures against a dark background. This control can be considered positive for:

    a *Legionella pneumophilia*
    b *Treponema pallidum*
    c *Candida albicans*
    d *Mycobacterium tuberculosis*

*467 A histochemical procedure for demonstrating nonspecific esterase will show the enzyme's:

   a structure
   b origin
   c activity
   d protein

*468 The tissue shown below is:

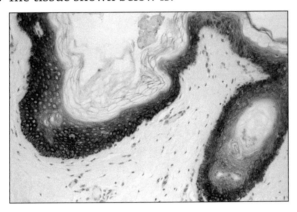

   a tonsil
   b esophagus
   c cervix
   d skin

*469 An H&E stained section is microscopically evaluated for quality. Which of the following is sufficient criterion for rejection of the slides?

   a crisp blue nuclei
   b pale pink to gray collagen
   c well defined chromatin
   d bright pink-red erythrocytes

*470 The terms acidophilic, basophilic, and sudanophilic reflect the ability of various cellular components to bind with:

   a eosin, phloxine, and Sudan IV
   b eosin, hematoxylin, and Sudan black B
   c hematoxylin, carmine, and oil red O
   d methyl green, hematoxylin, and Sudan III

*471 In the coupling method for alkaline phosphatase, the naphthol must be coupled with which of the following?

   a acetate
   b formazan
   c diazonium
   d phenylalanine

*472 The stain shown below would be LEAST useful in differentiating:

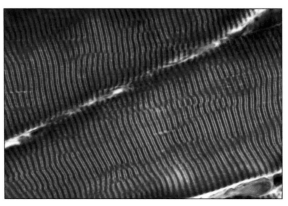

a fibrin
b rhabdomyosarcomas
c gliosis
d pheochromocytomas

*473 *Pneumocystis jirovecii* is BEST demonstrated by:

a hematoxylin and eosin
b periodic acid-Schiff
c methenamine silver
d Dieterle technique

*474 A control section used in a Grocott methenamine silver procedure is known to contain *Aspergillus* species. Microscopic evaluation reveals dense, black walls of the hyphae, with pale gray internal structures and a green background. This result should be considered:

a excellent
b minimally acceptable
c poor because the organisms are understained
d unacceptable because the wrong technique was used

*475 Consider the following staining results:

- PAS is negative
- alcian blue pH 2.5 is positive
- colloidal iron is positive

The stained sections most likely contain:

a neutral mucopolysaccharides
b basement membrane material
c fungal organisms
d acid mucopolysaccharides

*476 From one Z-line to the next in the image shown below is known as a/an:

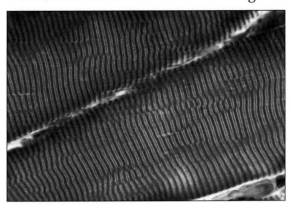

  a I-band
  b myofiliment
  c sarcomere
  d intercalated disc

*477 Just before use in the routine H&E procedure, acetic acid may be added to stock Harris hematoxylin to:

  a improve selectivity of the stain for chromatin
  b facilitate subsequent cytoplasmic staining
  c increase dye lake formation
  d avoid long bluing times

*478 The Schmorl technique depends upon:

  a ferric iron reduction
  b colloidal iron absorption
  c the argyrophil substance present
  d bilirubin oxidation

*479 Control material to be used with Best carmine technique can be found in the:

  a kidney
  b liver
  c testes
  d colon

*480 A section stained with Fouchet reagent shows discrete emerald-green globules. This indicates the presence of:

  a melanosomes
  b hemosiderin
  c bilirubin
  d acid hematin

*481 The differential diagnosis of a lymph node biopsy includes metastatic melanoma. Some tissue should be:

    a frozen for an enzyme profile
    b kept available for acid phosphatase demonstration
    c fixed for immunohistochemical staining with HMB-45 antibody
    d prepared for cytologic examination and fixed in Bouin fluid

*482 The blue stained material in the image below was stained with a/an:

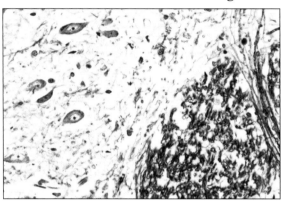

    a polychrome dye
    b iron hematoxylin lake
    c silver proteinate solution
    d sulfonated copper phthalocyanine dye

*483 A student submits a control section of small intestine on which a Schmorl stain has been done. No positive granules can be identified microscopically. Analysis of the procedure reveals the following:

    1 - ferric chloride and potassium ferrocyanide were used in the freshly prepared staining solution
    2 - the sections were stained for 7 minutes in each of 2 changes of the solution.

The problem can be identified as the fact that:

    a small intestine is not a good control for argentaffin cells
    b the staining solution should have contained potassium ferricyanide
    c the staining solution should have been aged
    d Schmorl technique does not demonstrate granules

*484 The microscopic quality control check of an H&E stained section reveals lightly stained nuclei lacking sharp chromatin detail. These results are an indication of:

    a poor fixation
    b poor processing
    c outdated bluing reagent
    d contaminated mountant

*485 DNA is NOT demonstrated on microscopic sections of a lymph node treated for 1 hour with 1 N hydrochloric acid at 60°C, followed by staining with Schiff reagent for 1 hour. The most likely explanation for this is:

    a the omission of a periodate oxidation step
    b excessive hydrolysis of the nuclei
    c the use of hydrochloric acid for pretreatment
    d excessive staining time in Schiff reagent

*486 In an immunoperoxidase procedure, the primary antibody used is a mouse monoclonal anti-Leu-4. Which secondary antibody would be appropriate?

    a goat anti-rabbit
    b goat anti-mouse
    c bovine serum albumin
    d biotinylated anti-rabbit

*487 In a Verhoeff-van Gieson stain, the tunica adventitia of large arteries stains similarly to:

    a elastin
    b epithelium
    c nuclei
    d collagen

*488 The structures stained blue-black in the image below most likely would NOT stain correctly if the:

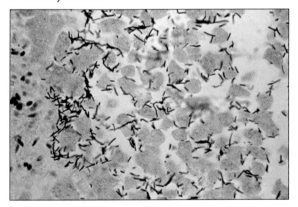

    a Brown and Brenn variant was used
    b picric acid solution could not be obtained
    c crystal violet was followed by iodine
    d patient was on antibotics

*489 The staining of fat by Sudan black B is due to the:

    a chemical linkage of fat and dye
    b adsorption of dye by fat
    c solubility of dye in fat
    d precipitation of dye in fat

*490 Refer to the following diagram:

$$NH^{3+}-\overset{\overset{\textstyle R}{|}}{\underset{\underset{\textstyle H}{|}}{C}}-COOH$$

The amphoteric amino acid shown in the above diagram:

    a migrates in an electrical field to the positive pole
    b is appropriately charged for eosin staining
    c is at the isoelectric point
    d is receptive to basic dyes

*491 One difference between rotary and linear automatic stainers is that rotary stainers:

    a require a different solution in each container
    b require the use of regressive dyes
    c permit different times in each compartment
    d permit staining of thicker sections

*492 The technique shown below will demonstrate sarcoplasmic reticulum, Z-band material and:

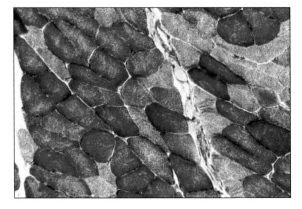

    a lysosomes
    b motor end-plates
    c mitochondria
    d euchromatin

*493 If you purchase an unlabeled monoclonal antibody to a specific antigen, the second antibody applied most commonly is:

    a rabbit anti-mouse
    b rabbit anti-goat
    c goat anti-human
    d mouse anti-human

*494 Pyroninophilia indicates the presence of:

    a deoxyribonucleic acid
    b ribonucleic acid
    c ribonuclease
    d mitochondria

*495 The auxochrome is the group present in dyes that:

    a acts as an oxidizer
    b is associated with color
    c is responsible for forming ionic bonds
    d features double bonds involving carbon and/or nitrogen

*496 Simultaneous coupling is a technique used in:

    a acid mucopolysaccharide demonstration
    b immunofluorescence
    c enzyme histochemistry
    d electron microscopy

*497 The Color Index printed on the label of a stain bottle refers to the:

    a purity of the stain
    b percentage of the stain present
    c maximum absorption peak
    d standard identification number

*498 A staining reaction that depends upon ionization of both the dye and the material on which the dye is precipitated is termed:

    a mordant staining
    b indirect staining
    c absorption
    d adsorption

*499 The material stained red by the technique shown below is a:

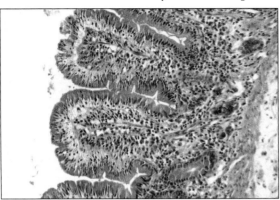

   a neutral mucin
   b sulfated mucin only
   c sulfated and carboxylated mucin
   d cellulose compound

*500 The naphthol AS-D chloroacetate esterase technique is useful in identifying which of the following cells?

   a fibroblasts
   b monocytes
   c granulocytes
   d lymphocytes

*501 Microscopic examination of a Carnoy fixed control section of kidney known to contain amyloid fails to show green birefringence following Congo red staining. This finding is:

   a correct for Congo red stains
   b indicative of a staining problem
   c the result of improper fixation
   d typical of freshly cut control sections

*502 Pure methyl green used at a slightly acid pH is considered a specific stain for:

   a aldehydes
   b polysaccharides
   c DNA
   d RNA

*503 The Weil stain will demonstrate which structure of the eye?

   a cornea
   b iris
   c optic nerve
   d sclera

*504 A false negative stain will most likely occur in the stain shown below if the tissue were fixed in:

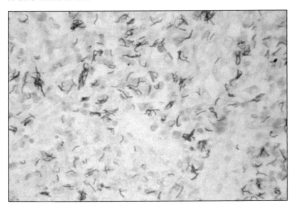

   a B-5 solution
   b Bouin solution
   c Carnoy solution
   d neutral buffered formalin

*505 The type of staining in which tissue soaks up dye and is completely penetrated by it is called:

   a adsorption
   b absorption
   c vital
   d routine

*506 The problem seen in the section shown below was most likely caused by:

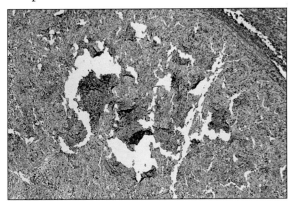

   a poor flotation bath practices
   b excessively vigorous epitope retrieval step
   c prolonged fixation of the tissue
   d the use of charged slides

*507 A bottle of a dye certified by the Biological Stain Commission:

   a shows the percentage by weight of the dye in the material
   b ensures that the material contains 100% dye by weight
   c has been assayed only for substances decolorized by titration with $TiCl_3$
   d is not evaluated for performance in a procedure

*508 Microscopic examination shows no pink staining on an H&E stained section. To isolate the problem, the first step is to:

   a repeat the dehydration step
   b recut and restain the sections
   c check the type of eosin
   d check the pH of the eosin

*509 The tissue shown below is often used as a control for this stain and can be identified as:

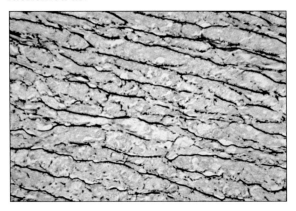

   a myometrium
   b aorta
   c muscular artery
   d adventitia

*510 The alcian blue, pH 2.5, stained slides consistently show blue staining of the nuclei. This could most likely be corrected by changing the procedure to include:

   a decreased time in the alcian blue solution
   b decreased hydration time during deparaffinization
   c rinsing with acetic acid after the alcian blue stain
   d increasing the temperature of the alcian blue staining

*511 An insulinoma is a neoplasm most commonly arises in the:

   a liver
   b thyroid
   c pituitary
   d pancreas

The following items have been identified as appropriate for both entry level histotechnicians and histotechnologists.

Answer Key–Staining

1	c	55	a	109	a	163	a	217	b	271	d
2	c	56	b	110	c	164	b	218	c	272	b
3	c	57	c	111	c	165	c	219	c	273	d
4	a	58	c	112	d	166	b	220	d	274	c
5	b	59	c	113	d	167	a	221	c	275	c
6	d	60	d	114	c	168	b	222	a	276	d
7	d	61	d	115	a	169	b	223	b	277	d
8	b	62	c	116	b	170	c	224	c	278	a
9	d	63	d	117	d	171	c	225	d	279	b
10	d	64	b	118	d	172	a	226	d	280	c
11	c	65	a	119	b	173	a	227	d	281	c
12	d	66	d	120	c	174	c	228	b	282	b
13	b	67	a	121	a	175	d	229	d	283	d
14	c	68	c	122	d	176	d	230	b	284	d
15	a	69	b	123	a	177	c	231	a	285	d
16	b	70	c	124	c	178	d	232	a	286	d
17	c	71	c	125	b	179	d	233	c	287	a
18	b	72	b	126	c	180	c	234	c	288	c
19	c	73	d	127	a	181	b	235	c	289	c
20	b	74	c	128	c	182	a	236	b	290	b
21	b	75	d	129	d	183	c	237	b	291	c
22	c	76	c	130	d	184	d	238	a	292	a
23	a	77	b	131	c	185	d	239	d	293	c
24	d	78	c	132	d	186	c	240	c	294	c
25	c	79	a	133	c	187	d	241	a	295	a
26	b	80	c	134	b	188	b	242	c	296	b
27	d	81	d	135	c	189	b	243	d	297	b
28	c	82	b	136	a	190	c	244	d	298	d
29	a	83	d	137	c	191	a	245	b	299	b
30	c	84	b	138	c	192	b	246	a	300	a
31	d	85	c	139	b	193	a	247	b	301	b
32	b	86	b	140	c	194	d	248	d	302	d
33	d	87	d	141	d	195	b	249	a	303	c
34	a	88	a	142	b	196	c	250	c	304	b
35	b	89	c	143	d	197	a	251	b	305	a
36	a	90	a	144	a	198	a	252	a	306	c
37	b	91	b	145	c	199	c	253	c	307	b
38	d	92	b	146	d	200	a	254	d	308	c
39	b	93	a	147	d	201	b	255	a	309	b
40	b	94	c	148	b	202	a	256	c	310	c
41	c	95	c	149	a	203	d	257	d	311	b
42	b	96	d	150	a	204	d	258	a	312	c
43	a	97	b	151	b	205	d	259	a	313	c
44	b	98	b	152	c	206	c	260	a	314	d
45	b	99	a	153	a	207	a	261	d	315	b
46	c	100	c	154	a	208	b	262	b		
47	d	101	a	155	c	209	d	263	c		
48	c	102	a	156	d	210	c	264	a		
49	c	103	a	157	c	211	a	265	b		
50	b	104	c	158	b	212	a	266	c		
51	d	105	d	159	c	213	d	267	c		
52	b	106	a	160	c	214	d	268	b		
53	c	107	c	161	d	215	c	269	c		
54	b	108	d	162	b	216	c	270	d		

ISBN 978-089189-6494 ©ASCP 2016

The following items (*) have been identified as more appropriate for entry level histotechnologists.

*316 c	*350 a	*384 d	*418 c	*452 d	*486 b
*317 b	*351 d	*385 c	*419 c	*453 a	*487 d
*318 b	*352 c	*386 b	*420 b	*454 b	*488 d
*319 c	*353 d	*387 d	*421 d	*455 a	*489 c
*320 d	*354 c	*388 d	*422 c	*456 a	*490 b
*321 b	*355 a	*389 c	*423 d	*457 c	*491 c
*322 c	*356 d	*390 d	*424 a	*458 b	*492 c
*323 c	*357 c	*391 c	*425 a	*459 a	*493 a
*324 a	*358 d	*392 c	*426 b	*460 d	*494 b
*325 a	*359 c	*393 b	*427 a	*461 b	*495 c
*326 d	*360 c	*394 c	*428 b	*462 c	*496 c
*327 d	*361 a	*395 d	*429 b	*463 c	*497 d
*328 c	*362 d	*396 a	*430 d	*464 a	*498 d
*329 a	*363 b	*397 c	*431 c	*465 b	*499 c
*330 c	*364 c	*398 d	*432 b	*466 d	*500 c
*331 c	*365 b	*399 a	*433 d	*467 c	*501 b
*332 d	*366 b	*400 b	*434 a	*468 d	*502 c
*333 b	*367 c	*401 d	*435 d	*469 b	*503 c
*334 a	*368 c	*402 d	*436 b	*470 b	*504 c
*335 c	*369 a	*403 d	*437 c	*471 c	*505 b
*336 c	*370 d	*404 b	*438 c	*472 d	*506 b
*337 d	*371 a	*405 b	*439 d	*473 c	*507 a
*338 a	*372 b	*406 c	*440 a	*474 a	*508 d
*339 a	*373 d	*407 d	*441 a	*475 d	*509 b
*340 b	*374 b	*408 c	*442 d	*476 c	*510 a
*341 b	*375 a	*409 a	*443 c	*477 a	*511 d
*342 d	*376 c	*410 b	*444 d	*478 a	
*343 c	*377 c	*411 c	*445 c	*479 b	
*344 a	*378 c	*412 a	*446 d	*480 c	
*345 d	*379 b	*413 c	*447 d	*481 c	
*346 b	*380 c	*414 c	*448 c	*482 d	
*347 b	*381 a	*415 c	*449 b	*483 b	
*348 c	*382 c	*416 a	*450 c	*484 a	
*349 b	*383 d	*417 d	*451 c	*485 b	

Answer Key–Staining

The following items have been identified as appropriate for both entry level histotechnicians and histotechnologists.

1   **c**   Mycobacteria are stained red by the Fite procedure. [Carson & Cappellano, p220]

2   **c**   Colloidal iron will bind to acid mucosubstances which may then be demonstrated by the Prussian blue reaction. [Carson & Cappellano, pp151-152]

3   **c**   Sites of glycogen removal will be demonstrated in the diastase section; whereas, glycogen will be retained and stained with the PAS reaction in the section without digestion. [Carson & Cappellano, pp141-142]

4   **a**   Formalin pigment is birefringent. [Carson & Cappellano, p11]

5   **b**   Acid mucosubstances may be differentiated from neutral mucosubstances by staining with both the alcian blue and PAS stains. Neutral mucins are positive with the PAS and negative with the alcian blue and acid mucosubstances are PAS negative and alcian blue positive. [Carson & Cappellano, p136]

6   **d**   The colloidal iron method is based on the formation of an ionic bond between ferric iron and the negatively charged carboxyl and sulfate groups of acid mucosubstances. [Bancroft & Gamble, p175]

7   **d**   Reticulin is demonstrated in the technique shown in the image. [Carson & Cappellano, pp174-177]

8   **b**   Sodium chloride is added to Congo red solutions to suppress background and nonspecific staining. [Carson & Cappellano, p155]

9   **d**   Acid mucosubstances exhibit metachromasia when stained with thionine, azure A, toluidine blue and other metachromatic dyes. [Bancroft & Gamble, p178]

10   **d**   The PAS reaction is useful for the demonstration of neutral mucosubstances. [Carson & Cappellano, pp138-139]

11   **c**   The preparation of van Gieson solution is critical for proper differentiation of muscle and collagen. If the picric acid is not saturated, collagen will not stain red and cytoplasm, muscle, and collagen may all stain the same color. [Carson & Cappellano, pp166, 168]

12   **d**   Slides must be rinsed well with water following staining in nuclear fast red or a cloudiness will develop over the entire slide that can be removed only by backing the slide up to water and washing well. [Carson & Cappellano, p176]

13   **b**   The black stained structures are fungi. [Carson & Cappellano, pp230-233]

14   **c**   Lipofuscin, a yellow-brown pigment, is frequently referred to as "wear and tear" pigment. It collects in the more permanent cells (eg, heart, liver, and neurons) of older persons, and in some disease states. [Carson & Cappellano, p243]

15   **a**   Hemosiderin, hemoglobin, and bile pigment are classified as endogenous, hematogenous pigments. [Carson & Cappellano, p242]

16   **b**   Iron hematoxylin is recommended for nuclear staining if it is to be followed by acidic solutions, as it will not be removed by acids. [Carson & Cappellano, p115]

17   **c**   The preferred thickness for the stain shown (Congo red) is 8 - 10 μm. [Carson & Cappellano, pp154-155]

18   **b**   Glial fibers can be demonstrated with a modified phosphotungstic acid hematoxylin procedure. [Carson & Cappellano, pp201-202]

19   **c**   The Grimelius stain is an argyrophil procedure, in that an external reducer is required to reduce the silver to a visible metallic form. [Carson & Cappellano, pp251-252]

20   **b**   Prolonged treatment with oxalic acid will ruin the silver proteinate reaction in the Bodian technique. [Carson & Cappellano, p193]

21   **b**   Fixation in Zenker solution will show increased eosin staining in muscle and red blood cells because Zenker does not bind to basic (cationic) cytoplasmic groups. [Carson & Cappellano, p22]

22   **c**   For immediate use, aluminum hematoxylin solutions must be chemically ripened. [Carson & Cappellano, pp112-113]

23   **a**   The image shown is a Masson trichrome stain. [Carson & Cappellano, pp162-163]

24   **d**   By varying the degree of differentiation and the solution pH, Nissl substance and nuclei can be preferentially stained. [Carson & Cappellano, p191]

25   **c**   Skeletal muscle fibers show cross-striations and multiple peripherally located nuclei. [Carson & Cappellano, p161]

26   **b**   The methyl green-pyronin technique for differentially staining nucleic acids (DNA: blue to blue-green, RNA: red) is shown. [Carson & Cappellano, pp127-129]

27   **d**   Light green is one of the counterstains used following some silver impregnation procedures, such as the Grocott methenamine silver nitrate fungus stain. [Carson & Cappellano, p233]

28   **c**   Melanin is one of the substances demonstrated by the Fontana-Masson technique. [Carson & Cappellano, pp248-249]

29   **a**   The Verhoeff-van Gieson stain is a regressive method for demonstrating elastic fibers, with differentiation by excess mordant. [Carson & Cappellano, pp167-168]

30   **c**   The differentiating solution in the Holzer method for glial fibers is aniline oil-chloroform. [Carson & Cappellano, pp202-203]

31   **d**   The technique shown is the von Kossa. [Carson & Cappellano, pp256-257]

32   **b**   The Feulgen stain can be used to demonstrate intracytoplasmic DNA-type viral inclusions in tissue; this stain is specific for DNA. [Carson & Cappellano, p126]

33   **d**   Propylene glycol is used in some oil red O and Sudan black B solutions to prevent the loss of lipids during the staining of fat. [Carson & Cappellano, p184]

Answers–Staining

34   **a**   For the best staining results, Verhoeff staining solution should be used for only a few hours because the ferric chloride in the solution is a strong oxidizing agent. [Carson & Cappellano, p167]

35   **b**   The Truant auramine-rhodamine is a very sensitive method for mycobacteria and good for verifying negative results that are expected to be positive. [Carson & Cappellano, pp221-222]

36   **a**   Schiff reagent that has been overused will give very pale unsatisfactory staining. [Carson & Cappellano, p1341]

37   **b**   Carnoy fixed tissue is preferred for the methyl green-pyronin stain unless the procedure has been modified for formalin fixed tissue. [Carson & Cappellano, pp128-129]

38   **d**   Hematoxylin, carmine, and orcein are natural dyes. [Carson & Cappellano, p111]

39   **b**   Melanin can be bleached by strong oxidizing agents, and potassium permanganate is one of the better reagents used for this purpose. [Bancroft & Gamble, p244]

40   **b**   The very alkalinity of the silver solutions, with a pH in the range of 11-12, will sometimes cause tissue to wash off slides, and it may be helpful to use special coated slides or charged slides. [Carson & Cappellano, p176]

41   **c**   The primary staining solution in the Schmorl technique contains ferric chloride and potassium ferricyanide. Reducing substances present in tissue reduce the ferric ions present in the solution to ferrous ions which immediately react with the ferricyanide present in the solution to form a precipitate known as Turnbull blue. [Carson & Cappellano, p247]

42   **b**   The stain shown is the Masson trichrome and the preferred fixative is Bouin solution. [Carson & Cappellano, p162]

43   **a**   The stain shown is the Verhoeff-van Gieson and the primary stain (Verhoeff solution) is made fresh each time before use. [Carson & Cappellano, p167]

44   **b**   With underdevelopment spirochetes are not seen or are only minimally stained. No oxidizer is used for staining spirochetes; the staining solution is heated to 54°C, and dirty glassware will cause a dirty background. [Brown, p80]

45   **b**   Argentaffin cells found in the stomach and intestines are known as enterochromaffin cells. [Kiernan, p426]

46   **c**   Staining is enhanced by the addition of both phenol and alcohol, and these reagents also aid in dissolving the basic fuchsin. [Carson & Cappellano, p216]

47   **d**   Ependymal cells are true epithelial cells lining the ventricles and the spinal canal. [Young & Lowe, p140]

48   **c**   Solutions of anionic dyes (eg, acid fuchsin) in picric acid are used to demonstrate both collagen and muscle. [Carson & Cappellano, p166]

49   **c**   Lipofuscin can be stained with Sudan black B and carbol-fuchsin. [Bancroft & Gamble, pp246-247]

50   **b**   Transitional epithelium refers to urothelium. [Young & Lowe, pp246-247]

51   **d**   The stain shown is the methyl green-pyronin and ribonucleic acid (RNA) is stained red. [Carson & Cappellano, p128-129]

52   **b**   The Verhoeff elastic stain performs well after any fixative, gives intense black staining of the elastic fibers, must be differentiated microscopically, and is a permanent stain that results in little fading. [Carson & Cappellano, pp167-168]

53   **c**   The material stained blue is collagen. The stain is the Masson trichrome. [Carson & Cappellano, p162]

54   **b**   Osmium tetroxide chemically combines with fat, blackening it in the process. Fat that has combined with osmium tetroxide is insoluble in alcohols and xylene, and the tissue can be processed for paraffin embedding. [Carson & Cappellano, p185]

55   **a**   The most common reducing agent used in diamine silver reticulin methods is formaldehyde. [Carson & Cappellano, p173]

56   **b**   The basic component of the central nervous system is the neuron. [Carson & Cappellano, p190]

57   **c**   The Luxol fast blue combined with the Holmes technique will demonstrate both axons and the myelin sheath. [Carson & Cappellano, pp209-210]

58   **c**   The technique shown is the Verhoeff-van Gieson. [Carson & Cappellano, pp167-168]

59   **c**   The Grocott methenamine silver is the most reliable technique for staining fungi in tissue. [Carson & Cappellano, pp229-232]

60   **d**   In addition to hematoxylin and potassium or ammonium aluminum sulfate, Mayer hematoxylin contains sodium iodate, chloral hydrate, and citric acid. [Carson & Cappellano, p114]

61   **d**   Most fungi are inconspicuous with the H&E stain and require special techniques that employ oxidation of the polysaccharides in the cell wall for demonstration. [Carson & Cappellano, pp226-234]

62   **c**   The hematoxylin and eosin (H&E) stain is most suitable for demonstrating general tissue morphology. [Bancroft & Gamble, p121]

63   **d**   Carbon is an exogenous pigment. [Carson & Cappellano, p242]

64   **b**   The silver techniques for reticulin employ the same major steps of oxidation, sensitization, impregnation, and reduction. [Carson & Cappellano, p173]

65   **a**   Birefringence of Congo red stained amyloid is demonstrated with polarizing microscopy in the image shown. [Carson & Cappellano, p155]

66   **d**   The cerebrum is the largest portion of the brain. [Young & Lowe, pp392, 399]

67 **a** Hemosiderin laden macrophages can be distinguished from other pigmented macrophages by the Prussian blue reaction. [Carson & Cappellano, pp245-246]

68 **c** Lipofuscin is commonly known as the "wear and tear" pigment. [Carson & Cappellano, p243]

69 **b** Bone is classified as either cancellous or compact. [Young & Lowe, pp192, 194]

70 **c** Melanin is normally found in the skin, hair, retina, iris, and certain parts of the central nervous system. [Carson & Cappellano, p243]

71 **c** If the background structures are an intense red in the Gram stain, it means that the picric acid-acetone differentiation was poor. [Carson & Cappellano, pp222-224]

72 **b** Aluminum hematoxylins are most commonly differentiated with hydrochloric acid in an alcoholic solution. [Carson & Cappellano, p111]

73 **d** The material stained purple in the large cells is Nissl substance. [Carson & Cappellano, pp190, 208

74 **c** Toludine blue is a metachromatic stain used for identifying mast cells. [Carson & Cappellano, p186]

75 **d** Connective tissue proper refers to collagen, reticulin, and elastin and also some connective tissue cells such as fibroblasts, fat cells, etc. [Carson & Cappellano, p160]

76 **c** The fibers stained purple are elastic fibers. [Carson & Cappellano, pp169-170]

77 **b** The iodine forms a dye-complex with crystal violet in the Gram stain. [Carson & Cappellano, p222]

78 **c** Squamous, cuboidal, and columnar are descriptive of different epithelial cells. [Young & Lowe, pp82-86]

79 **a** The group in a dye that confers color is called a chromophore. [Carson & Cappellano, p110]

80 **c** Hydroquinone is used in the Bodian stain. [Carson & Cappellano, pp193-194]

81 **d** The stain shown is the Feulgen reaction for DNA. [Carson & Cappellano, pp126-127]

82 **b** Differences in cell walls are primarily responsible for whether organisms stain Gram positive or Gram negative. [Carson & Cappellano, pp204-206]

83 **d** Ferric ammonium sulfate is used as the oxidizer and differentiator in the Weil stain for myelin. [Carson & Cappellano, pp204-206]

84 **b** Nuclear basophilia is impaired if tissue remains in Zenker fixative too long; fixation time should not exceed 24 hours. [Carson & Cappellano, p21]

85 **c** A Romanowsky type stain is the stain of choice for the differentiation of the different types of granulocytes. [Kiernan, pp178-180]

86 **b** Argentaffin substances have the ability to both bind silver and reduce it to its metallic form. [Carson & Cappellano, pxi]

87 **d** Sections that are not adequately dehydrated after the eosin will appear hazy and out of focus when examined microscopically; contrast between nucleus and cytoplasm will not be sharp. [Brown, p46]

ISBN 978-089189-6494 ©ASCP 2016

88   **a**   The cells stained blue are goblet cells. [Carson & Cappellano, p5; Young & Lowe, p84]

89   **c**   Mycobacteria are demonstrated with the auramine-rhodamine stain. [Carson & Cappellano, pp221-222]

90   **a**   The COOH group is an anionic auxochrome. [Carson & Cappellano, p110]

91   **b**   The bile pigment is converted to biliverdin in the Hall and Stein techniques. [Carson & Cappellano, p255]

92   **b**   Hydrochloric acid is used in the Prussian blue reaction. [Carson & Cappellano, p245]

93   **a**   The structures stained blue-black are Gram positive organisms. [Carson & Cappellano, p223]

94   **c**   Areolar connective tissue is also known as loose connective tissue. [Young & Lowe, p73]

95   **c**   Mayer hematoxylin is used only progressively. [Carson & Cappellano, p114]

96   **d**   If nuclei are stained red-brown to red, the hematoxylin is most likely overoxidized, or breaking down. [Brown, p44]

97   **b**   In the Hall method, bile is demonstrated by Fouchet reagent, which oxidizes bilirubin to biliverdin. [Carson & Cappellano, p255]

98   **b**   Paraldehyde used to prepare the aldehyde fuchsin stain should be fresh. [Carson & Cappellano, p171]

99   **a**   A problem will occur with the acid-fast techniques if the sections are allowed to dry after the carbol-fuchsin stain. [Carson & Cappellano, p217]

100   **c**   Excess adhesive on the slide may stain with eosin and cause a pink artifact surrounding the tissue and in the tissue spaces. [Carson & Cappellano, p73]

101   **a**   Muscle striations will stain blue with the PTAH stain. [Carson & Cappellano, pp178-179]

102   **a**   Muscle, collagen, and erythrocytes should stain different shades of pink with the H&E stain. [Carson & Cappellano, p116]

103   **a**   In the Gram stain, iodine should be applied after the crystal violet, forming a dye lake. [Carson & Cappellano, pp222-223]

104   **c**   Both the Gomori and Grocott techniques use a methenamine solution, Gomori in the demonstration of urates, and Grocott in the staining of fungi. [Carson & Cappellano, pp230-234, 254-255]

105   **d**   The tissue shown is skin. [Young & Lowe, p168]

106   **a**   Differential staining with the Giemsa solution is an example of polychromasia. [Carson & Cappellano, pp129-130]

107   **c**   Intercalated discs are unique to cardiac muscle. [Young & Lowe, pp 116-118, 153]

108   **d**   Artifactual pigments usually lie on the surface of cells and not within the cell; however formalin pigment has been reported within cell cytoplasm. [Carson & Cappellano, p242]

109 **a**   In the central nervous system, oligodendroglia function in the production and maintenance of the myelin sheaths surrounding axons. In the peripheral nervous system Schwann cells function in myelin production. [Carson & Cappellano, pp194-195]

110 **c**   Toluidine blue is an example of a metachromatic stain. [Carson & Cappellano, pp186-187]

111 **c**   Colloidal iron for acid mucosubstances is the technique shown. [Carson & Cappellano, pp151-153]

112 **d**   Most amoeba can be demonstrated with the periodic acid-Schiff procedure. [Bancroft & Gamble, p329]

113 **d**   Weigert hematoxylin is frequently used as a nuclear stain in special staining techniques. [Carson & Cappellano, p113]

114 **c**   The pigment formed by the reaction of ferrous ions with potassium ferricyanide is known as Turnbull blue. [Carson & Cappellano, p246]

115 **a**   The hematoxylin and eosin stain shown is not excellent because only 2 shades of eosin are apparent; an excellent stain would show 3 shades. [Carson & Cappellano, p116]

116 **b**   The dye alizarin red S will react with the calcium cations, forming an alizarin red S-calcium complex in a chelation process. [Carson & Cappellano, p257]

117 **d**   Mast cells contain granules that stain metachromatically. [Carson & Cappellano, p186]

118 **d**   The substance is amyloid, which will polarize apple green when stained with Congo red. [Carson & Cappellano, pp154-155]

119 **b**   Simple lipid stains are done on frozen sections as fat is soluble in the dehydrating and clearing agents used in paraffin processing procedures. [Carson & Cappellano, p185]

120 **c**   Collagen is the toughest of the connective tissue fibers. [Carson & Cappellano, p160; Young & Lowe, p66]

121 **a**   The only hematogenous pigment found in normal red blood cells is hemoglobin. [Carson & Cappellano, p242]

122 **d**   In the oil red O stain for fat, the dye is absorbed by the fat. The dye is more soluble in the fat than in the dye solvent. [Carson & Cappellano, p183]

123 **a**   The Schmorl technique depends upon the reduction of ferric ions to ferrous ions. The ferrous ions immediately combine with the ferricyanide present in the staining solution to form an insoluble blue precipitate (Turnbull blue). [Carson & Cappellano, p247]

124 **c**   The tissue shown is the small intestine. [Carson & Cappellano, p145; Young & Lowe, pp263, 274]

125 **b**   Elastic fibers stain violet-purple in the Gomori aldehyde fuchsin technique. [Carson & Cappellano, pp169-170]

126 **c**   Urate crystals may be demonstrated with a modified Gomori methenamine silver technique. [Carson & Cappellano, pp244, 254]

127 **a**   The Cajal gold sublimate technique will selectively stain astrocytes. [Carson & Cappellano, pp203-204]

128 **c** The Sevier-Munger will demonstrate both neurofibrils and neurosecretory granules. [Carson & Cappellano, pp199-200]

129 **d** Some argentaffin cells are also called endocrine cells, Kulchitsky cells, and enterochromaffin cells. [Young & Lowe, p282]

130 **d** The reticulin staining pattern is that typically seen in liver tissue. [Carson & Cappellano, p176]

131 **c** Ferric chloride is the differentiating solution in the Verhoeff-van Gieson procedure. [Carson & Cappellano, pp167-168]

132 **d** Impregnation methods involve selective deposition of a metallic substance on a tissue structure, and if necessary is then made visible by reduction of the metal. [Carson & Cappellano, p173]

133 **c** The periodic acid-Schiff technique will demonstrate *Entamoeba histolytica*. [Bancroft & Gamble, p329]

134 **b** Collagen stains green in the Gomori 1-step trichrome procedure. [Carson & Cappellano, p165]

135 **c** Nonkeratinizing stratified squamous lines the esophagus; keratinizing stratified squamous epithelium covers skin; transitional, or urothelium lines the bladder; ciliated pseudostratified columnar epithelium lines the trachea. [Young & Lowe, pp267-268]

136 **a** Mast cell granules stain well with toluidine blue. [Carson & Cappellano, pp186-187]

137 **c** Picric acid is contained in the counterstain of the technique shown (Verhoeff-van Gieson). [Carson & Cappellano, pp167-168]

138 **c** Chromaffin cells of the adrenal medulla are preserved only when fixed in a primary chromate fixative such as Orth. [Carson & Cappellano, p7]

139 **b** The stain is an acid-fast technique and the organisms are mycobacteria. [Carson & Cappellano, pp217-217]

140 **c** The basophilic material in the cytoplasm of neurons is rough endoplasmic reticulin with its content of RNA responsible for the basophilic staining. [Carson & Cappellano, p190]

141 **d** The Holmes technique is a modification of the Bodian technique. [Carson & Cappellano, p195]

142 **b** The Gram stain depends upon differences in the bacterial cell wall for differential staining. [Carson & Cappellano, p222]

143 **d** More uniform decolorization is achieved with alcoholic solutions of hydrochloric acid than with aqueous solutions. [Carson & Cappellano, p216]

144 **a** The periodic acid-Schiff stain is shown in the image and the technique depends upon the formation of aldehydes. [Carson & Cappellano, pp139-141]

Answers–Staining

145 **c** Gill hematoxylin contains ethylene glycol because it is an excellent solvent for hematoxylin and helps prevent the formation of surface precipitates, and it contains aluminum sulfate instead of the usual ammonium or potassium aluminum sulfate. [Carson & Cappellano, p114]

146 **d** The Steiner technique will demonstrate *Legionella pneumophila*. [Carson & Cappellano, pp238-239]

147 **d** Periodic acid is the oxidizer in the Jones and Gomori methenamine silver techniques for basement membranes. [Carson & Cappellano, pp180-182]

148 **b** False positive staining may occur with the periodic acid-Schiff stain on glutaraldehyde-fixed tissue due to an extra aldehyde group that may not be involved in protein crosslinking during fixation, but may be left free to react with the Schiff reagent. [Carson & Cappellano, p140]

149 **a** Formaldehyde is used as a reducer in the diamine silver methods for reticulin. [Carson & Cappellano, p173]

150 **a** Thionin and cresyl echt violet can be used to demonstrate Nissl substance [Carson & Cappellano, p190]

151 **b** The tissue shown in the image is small intestine. [Young & Lowe, p5]

152 **c** Uranyl acetate serves as a sensitizer in the Wilder reticulin procedure. [Carson & Cappellano, p173]

153 **a** On standing, most hematoxylin solutions will develop a metallic sheen of oxidized dye, actually aluminum-hematein, and the solution should be filtered before use or the precipitate can be picked up on the slides. [Brown, p45; Carson & Cappellano, p115]

154 **a** When connective tissue fibers and red cells are stained black with the GMS stain, it is most likely overexposure to hot methenamine silver solution. [Carson & Cappellano, p234]

155 **c** When microorganisms lie out of the focal plane of the tissue, it is most likely due to a contaminated staining solution or flotation bath. Most contaminants, or debris, will lie out of the focal plane of the section. [Brown, p62]

156 **d** The cells stained red-orange in the image shown are goblet cells. [Carson & Cappellano, pp5, 145]

157 **c** The stained structures are starch granules introduced by talcum powder from gloves of the pathologist or technologist; these granules can be easily identified by the characteristic Maltese cross configuration when polarized. [Bancroft & Gamble, p254]

158 **b** Spirochetes are argyrophilic and when impregnated with silver nitrate require an external reducing solution for visualization. [Carson & Cappellano, pp234-235]

159 **c** The milky xylene indicates that water is still present, so all dehydrating and clearing solutions should be changed. [Carson & Cappellano, p124]

160 **c** The cells shown are neurons and the purple granular material is Nissl substance. [Carson & Cappellano, p190]

161 **d** Celestine blue is the best substitute if hematoxylin is unavailable. [Carson & Cappellano, pp115-116]

162 **b** The PTAH is useful for demonstrating muscle striations. [Carson & Cappellano, pp178-179]

163 **a** Hemosiderin contains iron in the form of ferric hydroxide that is bound to a protein framework. [Bancroft & Gamble, p233]

164 **b** Collagen fibers vary from a regular arrangement to an irregular arrangement according to the location and function. [Carson & Cappellano, p160; Young & Lowe, p66]

165 **c** The red-brown nuclear staining most often is indicative of overoxidized hematoxylin, so the solution should be replaced with a new solution from another batch of hematoxylin. [Carson & Cappellano, p122]

166 **b** Chemically cleaned glassware should be used with silver impregnation methods, or a nonselective precipitation of silver may occur. [Brown, p91]

167 **a** Orcein in an acidified alcoholic solution stains elastic fibers brown; the resorcin-fuchsin and Verhoeff procedures stain elastic fibers black, and the aldehyde technique stains elastic fibers purple. [Carson & Cappellano, p170]

168 **b** Tissue fixed in Bouin solution will not give satisfactory results with the Feulgen technique because Bouin solution hydrolyzes the nuclei excessively during fixation. [Carson & Cappellano, p127]

169 **b** Liver tissue is the preferred control for the reticulin procedures. [Carson & Cappellano, p174]

170 **c** The sequence for the Feulgen reaction is hydrolysis with hydrochloric acid, reaction with Schiff reagent, then rinses with sulfurous acid to remove any unreacted Schiff reagent. [Carson & Cappellano, pp126-127]

171 **c** The precise preparation of the developing, or reducing, solution is critical and fresh reagents should be used in the preparation. [Brown, p80]

172 **a** Bouin solution functions as a mordant for the trichrome procedures. [Carson & Cappellano, pp162-165]

173 **a** Peanut oil is combined with xylene for deparaffinization of slides to be stained for the leprosy organism. This protects the waxy capsule of the organism and enhances acid-fastness. [Carson & Cappellano, pp220-221]

174 **c** The Schmorl technique can also be used to demonstrate melanin. [Carson & Cappellano, pp247-248]

175 **d** Iodine and ferric chloride serve as mordants in the Verhoeff-van Gieson technique, but they also have an oxidizing functions that assists in converting hematoxylin to hematein. [Carson & Cappellano, p167]

Answers–Staining

176 **d** Anthracotic, or carbon, pigment is often found in the lungs and hilar lymph nodes. It is insoluble in concentrated sulfuric acid, a characteristic that aids in differentiating it from melanin, formalin, and malarial pigments. [Carson & Cappellano, p242]

177 **c** Elastic fibers can be demonstrated by resorcin-fuchsin and orcein stains. [Carson & Cappellano, p170]

178 **d** If the sodium thiosulfate is omitted, unreduced silver will not be removed and nonspecifically bound silver remaining in the sections may be reduced later by exposure to light. [Carson & Cappellano, p173]

179 **d** The PAS stain is demonstrated and it stains neutral mucopolysaccharides; chondroitin sulfate and heparin are acid mucopolysaccharides. [Carson & Cappellano, p138]

180 **c** The mordants linking hematoxylin to tissue are generally classified as metallic. [Carson & Cappellano, p112]

181 **b** Phosphomolybdic acid is the oxidizer in the Wilder reticulin method. [Carson & Cappellano, p173]

182 **a** The technique shown is Mayer mucicarmine. [Carson & Cappellano, pp144-146]

183 **c** Potassium permanganate is the oxidizer in the Gomori reticulin method. [Carson & Cappellano, p173]

184 **d** Non-metallic forceps and chemically cleaned glassware are used in silver techniques to prevent contamination of the silver solution. [Carson & Cappellano, p175]

185 **d** The black stained structures are spirochetes. [Carson & Cappellano, p235]

186 **c** Adipocytes is another name for fat cells. [Young & Lowe, pp74-75]

187 **d** Elastic fibers have an affinity for orcein. [Carson & Cappellano, p170]

188 **b** Brown-Hopps is the preferred technique used to demonstrate Gram negative bacteria in tissue sections. [Carson & Cappellano, p223]

189 **b** A reticular fiber meshwork forms the supporting framework of organs such as spleen and lymph nodes. [Young & Lowe, p67]

190 **c** Chromic acid is used in the GMS procedure to oxidize polysaccharides to aldehydes. [Carson & Cappellano, p230]

191 **a** Copper is used in the Bodian technique to "destain" connective tissue; it is thought to replace the silver that has impregnated the connective tissue fibers. [Carson & Cappellano, p193]

192 **b** Mycosis is the term used to designate the disease produced by fungal organisms, as seen in the image. [Carson & Cappellano, p215]

193 **a** An azure-eosin is used in the Romanowsky type dye used in a rapid stain for *Helicobacter pylori*. [Carson & Cappellano, pp224-225]

194 **d**   EA solutions contain light green, eosin Y, and phosphotungstic acid. Some formulas also contain Bismarck brown. [Carson & Cappellano, pp326-327]

195 **b**   Antigen detection is improved in many cases by epitope retrieval, thus preventing a false negative result. [Carson & Cappellano, p268]

196 **c**   Hydrochloric acid is used for hydrolysis which results in the generation of aldehydes that can be demonstrated with Schiff reagent. [Carson & Cappellano, p126]

197 **a**   Silver is used in the method shown (von Kossa) to demonstrate calcium. [Carson & Cappellano, pp256-257]

198 **a**   Urates can be demonstrated with the Grocott methenamine silver method. [Carson & Cappellano, p254]

199 **c**   Avidin-biotin methods are used in immunohistochemical staining. [Carson & Cappellano, p271]

200 **a**   The Schmorl method stains reducing substances blue as a result of Turnbull blue formation. [Carson & Cappellano, pp246-247]

201 **b**   The oxidizer in the technique shown (PAS) is periodic acid. [Carson & Cappellano, p139]

202 **a**   The pH of the staining solution is critical for the Romanowsky-type stains and ideally should be adjusted for different fixatives. [Carson & Cappellano, p131]

203 **d**   Chromatin, specifically heterochromatin stains strongly with basic dyes. [Carson & Cappellano, p107]

204 **d**   Axons carry electrical impulses away from the neuron cell body. [Carson & Cappellano, p190]

205 **d**   Luxol fast blue stains are differentiated by lithium carbonate and 70% alcohol. [Carson & Cappellano, p206]

206 **c**   The method shown is for iron and it uses hydrochloric acid and potassium ferrocyanide. [Carson & Cappellano, p254]

207 **a**   Muscle fibers stain red in the Masson trichrome technique. [Carson & Cappellano, pp162-163]

208 **b**   The rhodanine method is the most sensitive of the techniques for detecting the presence of copper in tissue. [Carson & Cappellano, p272]

209 **d**   Antigens are molecules made up of proteins, carbohydrates, or other polymers, and are capable of producing an immune response in animals. [Carson & Cappellano, p264]

210 **c**   Potassium permanganate functions as an oxidizer. [Carson & Cappellano, pp173, 178]

211 **a**   The organisms stain black with silver because of the subsequent application of a chemical reducing agent; the method used is an argyrophil technique. [Carson & Cappellano, pp234-235]

212 **a**   The dye solution most commonly used for staining *Mycobacterium tuberculosis* is composed of basic fuchsin and phenol. [Carson & Cappellano, p216]

213 **d**   Ammonia water, lithium carbonate solution, and Scott tap water substitute are examples of bluing agents. [Carson & Cappellano, p115]

Answers–Staining

214 **d** The black stained structures are known as hyphae. [Carson & Cappellano, pp215-231]

215 **c** The second cytoplasmic stain in the Papanicolaou method is some type of EA, which is a polychrome stain containing eosin Y, light green yellowish SF, and possibly Bismarck brown. [Carson & Cappellano, pp326-327]

216 **c** Gallego is one of the differentiating solutions in the Brown-Hopps stain. [Carson & Cappellano, pp222-223]

217 **b** Elastic fibers stain blue-black to black in the Verhoeff-van Gieson technique. [Carson & Cappellano, pp167-168]

218 **c** Hydroquinone is the most commonly used chemical for reducing absorbed silver to a visible metallic stain in argyrophil procedures. [Carson & Cappellano, pp234-239]

219 **c** The blue-black structures are Gram positive bacilli. [Carson & Cappellano, p223]

220 **d** The term "argentaffin" literally denotes a reaction wherein cells have the ability to bind or be impregnated with silver and to reduce it to its metallic form. [Carson & Cappellano, pxi]

221 **c** Melanin pigment can be bleached with potassium permanganate; melanin is insoluble in most organic solvents or in anything that will significantly destroy the tissue that contains it. [Bancroft & Gamble, p244; Carson & Cappellano, p243]

222 **a** More selective nuclear staining can be achieved by adding either an excess of aluminum or an excess of acid. An excess of aluminum will counteract overoxidation by chemical oxidizers, and an excess of acid will provide H^+ to combine with weakly acidic groups in the tissue sections and prevent them from taking up hematoxylin. [Carson & Cappellano, p113]

223 **b** If the mounting medium has become too thick from evaporation of the solvent, the cover glass may be held too far above the section. This will cause microscopic problems. [Carson & Cappellano, p132]

224 **c** Prolonged storage of cut control slides for the Congo red stain will cause a loss of positivity. [Carson & Cappellano, p154]

225 **d** Hyphae are associated with some types of fungi. [Carson & Cappellano, p215]

226 **d** Lambda is a light chain present in some antibodies. [Carson & Cappellano, p254]

227 **d** Cancellous bone is composed of a network of bony trabeculae separated by interconnecting bone marrow spaces. [Young & Lowe, p195]

228 **b** The tissue shown in the image is skin. [Carson & Cappellano, p249]

229 **d** Potassium permanganate is the oxidizer in both the Snook and the Laidlaw reticulin procedures. [Carson & Cappellano, p173]

230 **b** The second differentiating solution used in the Weil method contains sodium borate and potassium ferricyanide. [Carson & Cappellano, p204]

231 **a** The acid-fastness of some organisms appears to be related to the lipid content of their wall. [Carson & Cappellano, p216]

232 **a** Increasing the temperature of the dye solution will increase the diffusion rate of the dye molecules, possibly by swelling the tissue components. [Carson & Cappellano, p111]

233 **c** Mayer mucicarmine can also be used to demonstrate *Cryptococcus neoformans*. [Carson & Cappellano, p146]

234 **c** Adipose cells are sudanophilic. [Bancroft & Gamble, p192; Carson & Cappellano, pp160,184]

235 **c** Alkaline phosphatase is used as the enzyme label in some immunohistochemical methods. [Carson & Cappellano, p269]

236 **b** In the von Kossa technique for calcium, the sections are placed in silver nitrate solution, and the solution is exposed to bright sunlight. [Carson & Cappellano, p256]

237 **b** Glial fibers are stained with crystal violet in the Holzer technique. [Carson & Cappellano, pp202-203]

238 **a** The nuclei are stained with Schiff reagent in the Feulgen reaction. [Carson & Cappellano, pp126-127]

239 **d** The organisms are mycobacteria which can also be demonstrated with auramine-rhodamine. [Carson & Cappellano, pp221-222]

240 **c** Phosphomolybdic-phosphotungstic acid is the differentiating solution that follows acid fuchsin-Biebrich scarlet in the Masson technique. This removes stain from collagen. [Carson & Cappellano, pp162-163]

241 **a** Elastic fibers seen in the image are stained black by iron hematoxylin. [Carson & Cappellano, pp167-168]

242 **c** Nissl substance is composed primarily of rough endoplasmic reticulum. [Carson & Cappellano, p190]

243 **d** In the PAP method of antigen detection, the PAP complex is made in the same species as the primary antibody. [Carson & Cappellano, p287]

244 **d** The black stained structures are fungi and they can also be demonstrated with the periodic acid-Schiff technique. [Carson & Cappellano, pp226, 231]

245 **b** Aldehyde fuchsin is stable for 3 to 4 weeks if stored at 4°C. [Bancroft & Gamble, p154; Carson & Cappellano, p171]

246 **a** The Luxol fast blue combined with the PAS demonstrates the myelin sheath, basement membranes, senile plaques, fungi, and corpora amylacea. It allows a correlative study of the cellular elements, fiber pathways, and vascular components of the nervous system. [Carson & Cappellano, pp210-211]

247 **b** Rosaniline (CI 42510) should not be used for the preparation of aldehyde fuchsin; pararosaniline (CI 42500) should be used. [Carson & Cappellano, p170]

248 **d** Calcium is not stained by the argentaffin procedures; melanin, enterochromaffin cells (argentaffin cells), and formalin pigment will stain. [Carson & Cappellano, pp248-249, 256-257]

©ASCP 2016   ISBN 978-089189-6494

Answers–Staining

249 **a** Ferric ferrocyanide is the end product of the iron stain. [Carson & Cappellano, p245]

250 **c** Schiff reagent is sometimes referred to as leucofuchsin because of the reduction of basic fuchsin to a colorless compound. The reaction described is the PAS stain. [Carson & Cappellano, p139]

251 **b** Chromatolysis refers to the loss of Nissl substance. [Carson & Cappellano, p190]

252 **a** Argentaffin is the term that describes the ability to bind and reduce silver without the use of a separate reducing agent. [Carson & Cappellano, p248]

253 **c** Gold chloride is used in the silver impregnation methods as a toner. [Carson & Cappellano, p173]

254 **d** The silvery-white birefringent material in the upper right corner is collagen. [Carson & Cappellano, pp55, 160]

255 **a** The Movat pentachrome stain will distinguish muscle, elastic fibers, collagen, fibrin, and mucin. [Carson & Cappellano, pp171-172]

256 **c** The technique shown (PAS) can also be used to stain glycogen. [Carson & Cappellano, pp141-142]

257 **d** Fibroblasts are the cells responsible for the production of connective tissue fibers (extracellular, nonliving elements). [Carson & Cappellano, p160]

258 **a** The melanin-containing cells are found in the epidermis. [Young & Lowe, pp172-173]

259 **a** Complete decolorization of the organisms will result if repeated attempts to remove the insoluble compound are made after the carbol-fuchsin has dried on the slide and the insoluble compound has formed. [Carson & Cappellano, p217]

260 **a** Microincineration involves burning off the organic content of tissue, leaving only the inorganic content remaining. [Carson & Cappellano, p244]

261 **d** Sections should not be allowed to dry at any stage of the Brown-Hopps procedure, or insoluble compounds that are difficult, if not impossible, to remove may be formed. [Carson & Cappellano, p224]

262 **b** Potassium permanganate and phosphomolybdic acid function as oxidizers in the methods for reticulin. [Carson & Cappellano, p173]

263 **c** Myelin is stained by the Luxol fast blue method. [Carson & Cappellano, pp206-207]

264 **a** Potassium permanganate can be used to ripen phosphotungstic acid –hematoxylin for immediate use. [Carson & Cappellano, p178]

265 **b** The staining of simple fat depends on the solubility of the dye in the lipid; the dye must be more soluble in the lipid than in the usual hydroalcoholic dye solvent. This a physical method of staining. [Carson & Cappellano, p183]

ISBN 978-089189-6494 ©ASCP 2016

266 **c** Collagen and muscle may be difficult to distinguish morphologically and the Masson trichrome is frequently used to distinguish between them in tumors. [Carson & Cappellano, p162]

267 **c** Small amounts of iron are normally found in the spleen. [Carson & Cappellano, p245]

268 **b** The black stained structures (spirochetes) are most likely stained with the Steiner procedure. [Carson & Cappellano, pp238-239]

269 **c** Regressive staining with hematoxylin involves overstaining and then decolorizing with dilute hydrochloric acid to the desired intensity. [Carson & Cappellano, p115]

270 **d** A combination of derivatives of methylene blue and eosin provide the color range of Romanowsky stains. [Carson & Cappellano, p129]

271 **d** The crystal violet stain for the demonstration of amyloid does not yield permanent preparations. [Carson & Cappellano, p156]

272 **b** The absence of red staining of epithelial cells and smooth muscle around the blood vessels indicate a depleted or old stain. [Carson & Cappellano, p164]

273 **d** Tissue for PTAH staining that has been fixed in formalin should be mordanted in either Zenker or Bouin solution. The PTAH stain should be aged; washing well after staining will cause a loss of the red-brown color; and sections should be cut at 4 - 5 μm. [Carson & Cappellano, pp178-179]

274 **c** A sharp differentiation between gray and white matter will be seen on a good Luxol fast blue stain. [Carson & Cappellano, p206]

275 **c** Thioflavin T is another method that can be used to demonstrate the component stained green (amyloid). [Carson & Cappellano, p157]

276 **d** The best PTAH staining solution is one that is allowed to ripen naturally. [Carson & Cappellano, p178]

277 **d** *Mycobacterium tuberculosis* may be demonstrated with carbol-fuchsin. [Carson & Cappellano, pp214, 216]

278 **a** Synthetic resins are hydrophobic; they do not tolerate water. [Carson & Cappellano, pp132-133]

279 **b** The technique shown is used to demonstrate hemosiderin. [Carson & Cappellano, p245]

280 **c** Spirochetes in fixed tissue are best demonstrated by metallic impregnation. [Carson & Cappellano, pp234-239]

281 **c** Sections stained with oil-soluble dyes (eg, fat stains) must be mounted with a medium that will not dissolve the lipids. [Carson & Cappellano, p184]

282 **b** Fite, Ziehl-Neelsen, and Kinyoun are names associated with microorganisms, specifically acid-fast bacteria. [Carson & Cappellano, pp216-220]

283 **d** In the Feulgen reactions, hydrochloric acid reacts with DNA to create aldehyde groups. [Carson & Cappellano, p126]

284 **d** Colon is a good control for the alcian blue technique, pH 2.5. [Carson & Cappellano, p147]

Answers–Staining

285 **d** The technique shown (Fontana-Masson) may be used to demonstrate argentaffin cells. [Carson & Cappellano, p248]

286 **d** The solution must be agitated at some point when the microwave oven is used for staining, or the section at the top of the slide will not stain at the same rate as the section at the bottom because of uneven heating of the solution. [Carson & Cappellano, pp67-68]

287 **a** Diastase is used to remove glycogen from cells in the PAS stain. [Carson & Cappellano, pp141-142]

288 **c** Nissl substance is demonstrated by the Luxol fast blue-cresyl echt violet stain. [Carson & Cappellano, pp207-208]

289 **c** The colloidal iron stain may be used instead of the alcian blue technique, pH 2.5, although it is not considered as specific for acid mucosubstances. [Carson & Cappellano, pp151-153]

290 **b** The technique shown is the Luxol fast blue. [Carson & Cappellano, pp206-207]

291 **c** Borax ferricyanide differentiates the Weil stain by oxidation. [Carson & Cappellano, p204]

292 **a** Regressive staining involves first overstaining the desired element and then differentiating. [Carson & Cappellano, pxvi]

293 **c** The PAS may be used to stain glycogen, neutral polysaccharides, and some glycoproteins. [Carson & Cappellano, pp139-140]

294 **c** Poor results might be obtained with the technique shown (Warthin-Starry), as well as other silver stains, if the glassware used was not chemically cleaned. [Carson & Cappellano, pp175, 234-235]

295 **a** Iron will be stained with a solution containing equal parts of 2% solutions of potassium ferrocyanide and hydrochloric acid. [Carson & Cappellano, p245]

296 **b** Bouin fixed tissue is unsatisfactory for the Feulgen reaction. [Carson & Cappellano, pp126-127]

297 **b** The Bodian stain is used to demonstrate axons and other nerve fibers. [Carson & Cappellano, p193]

298 **d** A dye lake is formed when a dye is combined with a mordant. [Carson & Cappellano, p112]

299 **b** Delafield hematoxylin is commonly aged with light. [Carson & Cappellano, p113]

300 **a** The technique shown (Mayer mucicarmine) is used for the demonstration of acid mucosubstances. [Carson & Cappellano, p144]

301 **b** Acid dyes are generally differentiated in solutions that are weakly basic; for example, eosin can be removed by a weak solution of ammonia. [Carson & Cappellano, p111]

302 **d** An amphoteric substance is one that can act as either an acid or a base, depending on the pH of the solution. [Carson & Cappellano, pxi]

303   **c**   The substance stained in the image shown is a neutral mucosubstance. The PAS stains neutral mucosubstances. [Carson & Cappellano, pp139-140]

304   **b**   The loss of basophilia may be caused by prolonged storage of wet tissue in unbuffered formalin. [Carson & Cappellano, p120]

305   **a**   If the neutralizing solution is not well washed out, the tissue is left slightly basic and the basic proteins are not appropriately charged for eosin uptake. [Brown, p41; Carson & Cappellano, p119]

306   **c**   Adsorption is the accumulation of stain by the surface of a tissue component. [Carson & Cappellano, pxi]

307   **b**   Weigert hematoxylin solution is generally unsatisfactory for use after 3 to 4 days. [Carson & Cappellano, p115]

308   **c**   Epithelium should stain red with the Masson trichrome. [Carson & Cappellano, pp162-164]

309   **b**   The milky appearance of slides when put in xylene prior to coverslipping indicates the presence of water and that adequate dehydration has not occurred. [Carson & Cappellano, p124]

310   **c**   If the slides are allowed to stay in the differentiating solution following the hematoxylin, the nuclear stain will most likely be too pale. [Carson & Cappellano, p122]

311   **b**   Dyes used for nuclear staining are basic. [Carson & Cappellano, p109]

312   **c**   Hematoxylin solutions must be oxidized to be effective stains. [Carson & Cappellano, p112]

313   **c**   The Verhoeff-van Gieson stain is overdifferentiated. [Carson & Cappellano, pp167-168]

314   **d**   Epitopes are antigenic determinants present on complete antigenic molecules. [Carson & Cappellano, pxiii]

315   **b**   Fluorochromes are dyes that absorb light and then emit light at a longer wavelength. [Carson & Cappellano, pp56, 269]

The following items (*) have been identified as more appropriate for entry level histotechnologists.

*316   **c**   *Cryptococcus neoformans* is a fungus that can be demonstrated by acidic mucin stains such as mucicarmine and alcian blue. [Carson & Cappellano, p145]

*317   **b**   If problems in differentiation occur, different pHs should be tried. [Carson & Cappellano, p305]

*318   **b**   Hemochromatosis is a pathologic condition in which too much iron is stored. This can result from multiple transfusions, increased dietary consumption, hemolysis, and severe congestion. [Carson & Cappellano, p245]

*319   **c**   No mucin containing structures (eg, goblet cells) are present to demonstrate the acid mucins; the tissue is very autolyzed and should not have been selected for this stain. [Carson & Cappellano, p147]

*320   **d**   Alpha-naphthyl acetate esterase will demonstrate denervated muscle fibers and motor end plates. [Carson & Cappellano, pp301-302]

*321 **b**   The Diff-Quik is the most rapid technique for *Helicobacter pylori*; the silver techniques require much more time. [Carson & Cappellano, pp224-225, 234-239]

*322 **c**   Acid phosphatase is considered a marker for lysosomes; the acid phosphatase stain indicates the presence of inflammatory cells in the tissue. [Carson & Cappellano, p306]

*323 **c**   The final colored product in the PAS reaction is achieved by restoration of the quinoid structure. [Carson & Cappellano, p139]

*324 **a**   The mucicarmine technique is specific for mucins of epithelial origin, so the technique may be useful for the identification of adenocarcinomas. [Bancroft & Gamble, p174]

*325 **a**   The naphthol AS-D chloroacetate esterase is one of the rare enzyme techniques that can be performed on paraffin sections. [Carson & Cappellano, p302]

*326 **d**   The activity of succinic dehydrogenase will be destroyed by fixation, as will the activity of many enzymes. [Carson & Cappellano, pp296, 310]

*327 **d**   The final reaction product in the technique shown (ATPase) is cobalt sulfide. [Carson & Cappellano, pp303-304]

*328 **c**   Acid phosphatase falls under the hydrolases. [Carson & Cappellano, pp297, 306]

*329 **a**   Cofactors are nonprotein structures that speed up the rate of enzyme reactions [Carson & Cappellano, p295]

*330 **c**   Enzymes that catalyze chemical reactions in biologic systems are proteins. [Carson & Cappellano, p295]

*331 **c**   The Grimelius stain will demonstrate carcinoid tumors as well as alpha cells of the pancreas. [Bancroft & Gamble, p286; Carson & Cappellano, p252]

*332 **d**   A negative phosphorylase stain indicates a phosphorylase deficiency in McArdle disease. [Carson & Cappellano, pp311-312]

*333 **b**   The spirochetes seen in the image are most likely *Treponema pallidum*. [Carson & Cappellano, pp214,234-235]

*334 **a**   The *Mycobacterium tuberculosis* organisms possess a fatty capsule containing a long-chain fatty acid (mycolic acid). [Bancroft & Gamble, p314]

*335 **c**   The most frequently used antibody in immunohistochemistry is IgG. [Bancroft & Gamble, p435]

*336 **c**   Reddish-brown nuclear staining may result when the hematoxylin is breaking down. [Carson & Cappellano, p122]

*337 **d**   Pretreating with nonimmune serum from the same animal species as the secondary antibody will reduce background staining. [Carson & Cappellano, p276]

*338 **a**   The brown stained structure is the epithelium. [Young & Lowe, p86]

*339 **a**   Compounds and tissue elements that fluoresce naturally have the property of autofluoresence. [Carson & Cappellano, p56]

ISBN 978-089189-6494   ©ASCP 2016

*340 **b** *Candida albicans* can appear as a mixture of budding yeast cells and pseudohypha elements. [Carson & Cappellano, p215]

*341 **b** Systemic mycoses go beyond superficial or cutaneous involvement to affect vital organs and cause extensive disease and even death. The incidence of systemic mycoses has increased because of the increase in the number of patients with compromised immune systems. [Bancroft & Gamble, p320]

*342 **d** A section from the medulla is shown in the image. [Carson & Cappellano, p207]

*343 **c** The Bielschowsky stain is useful for demonstrating the senile plaques and neurofibrillary tangles seen in Alzheimer disease. [Carson & Cappellano, pp196-197]

*344 **a** The NADH is an dehydrogenase enzyme procedure that demonstrates more positive staining in type I muscle fibers than in in type II fibers. [Carson & Cappellano, pp308-309]

*345 **d** An orthochromatic dye stains tissue the color of the dye itself. [Carson & Cappellano, pxv]

*346 **b** The nonspecific background stain in the image most likely resulted from a primary antibody that was too concentrated. [Brown, pp144-145]

*347 **b** Rickettsial organisms sometimes stain with the Giemsa technique, although they rarely need to be demonstrated in tissue sections. [Bancroft & Gamble, p324]

*348 **c** Only mitochondria are stained with the succinic dehydrogenase technique. The NADH diaphorase technique will demonstrate mitochondria, Z-band material, and sarcoplasmic reticulum. [Carson & Cappellano, p310]

*349 **b** A section from a carcinoma provides a good control for the Cam 5.2 antibody. [Carson & Cappellano, p277]

*350 **a** The phosphotungstic acid-hematoxylin stain is the nonimmunohistochemical stain used to aid in making a definitive diagnosis of rhabdomyosarcoma. [Carson & Cappellano, pp178-179]

*351 **d** The Masson trichrome stain is often used in making a diagnosis of cirrhosis of the liver. [Carson & Cappellano, p162]

*352 **c** Coated asbestos fibers can be made more visible by staining with the Prussian blue reaction. [Carson & Cappellano, p242]

*353 **d** Plasma cells are responsible for the production of immunoglobulins. [Carson & Cappellano, p160]

*354 **c** Melanosis coli pigment is a reducing substance and will give a positive reaction with the Schmorl technique. [Bancroft & Gamble, p248]

*355 **a** If the cresyl echt violet is not properly acidified, the background will be stained diffusedly and differentiation of the Nissl substance and cell nuclei will be impossible to detect. [Carson & Cappellano, p208]

*356 **d** Astrocytes can be demonstrated by using the antibody that is specific for GFAP. [Bancroft & Gamble, p381]

*357 c The variable regions are the combining sites of antibody molecules. [Kiernan, p485]

*358 d Melanin can be bleached by all of the listed chemicals except acetone. [Bancroft & Gamble, p244]

*359 c The ATPase stain shown is a metallic precipitation technique. [Carson & Cappellano, pp303-304]

*360 c The Mallory PTAH technique demonstrates the loss of muscle striations. [Carson & Cappellano, pp178-179]

*361 a Skin is a good control for the AE1/AE3 cytokeratin antibody as the epithelium will be stained. The other antibodies listed are for leukocytes. [Young & Lowe, p82]

*362 d Ground substance is the gel-like material that forms the bulk of extracellular content in connective tissue. [Young & Lowe, p65]

*363 b Negri bodies are small cell inclusions found in the brain of patients with rabies; they are one of the rare viral cytoplasmic inclusions that can be seen with the light microscope. [Carson & Cappellano, p215]

*364 c In the PAP method of staining, the PAP complex should be prepared in the same animal species as the primary antibody; this allows the secondary antibody to link to both the primary antibody and the PAP complex. [Carson & Cappellano, p287]

*365 b Argentaffin cells of the gastrointestinal tract are components of the amine uptake and carboxylase (APUD) system and tumors arising from these cells may be called apudomas. [Bancroft & Gamble, pp283-284]

*366 b Cryptococcosis is a disease characterized by narrow-based budding, carminophilic yeast cells. [Carson & Cappellano, p215]

*367 c Starch in introduced into tissues by talcum powder from the gloves of surgeons, nurses, or pathologists. When polarized it will produce a Maltese cross configuration. [Bancroft & Gamble, p254]

*368 c The malarial pigment that occurs in *Plasmodium* parasites is closely related to formalin pigment. [Bancroft & Gamble, p253; Carson & Cappellano, p242]

*369 a A solution of hydrogen peroxide in methanol is used to block endogenous peroxidase in immunohistochemical reactions using horseradish peroxidase. [Carson & Cappellano, p274]

*370 d Luxol fast blue dye has a structural formula closely related to that of alcian blue. [Carson & Cappellano, p206]

*371 a The stain shown is the NADH diaphorase. [Carson & Cappellano, pp308-309]

*372 b The antigen retrieval or epitope enhancement methods, including heat induced epitope retrieval (HIER) enhance primary staining and decrease background staining. Some antigens do not need HIER or EIER for demonstration. [Carson & Cappellano, p268]

ISBN 978-089189-6494 ©ASCP 2016

*373 **d** One possible cause of the poor staining is not mordanting formalin fixed tissue in Bouin solution; therefore, the stain should be repeated on another section. If the tissue was mordanted, then other possible causes should be identified. [Carson & Cappellano, p164]

*374 **b** When both the positive control and the specimen show weak staining, the most likely cause is incorrectly done epitope retrieval. [Carson & Cappellano, p268]

*375 **a** *Cryptosporidium* is one of a group of protozoa that causes severe and relentless outbreaks of diarrhea among AIDS patients. [Bancroft & Gamble, p330]

*376 **c** The artifact is known as corn flaking and is caused by letting the slides dry before applying the mounting medium and cover glass. [Carson & Cappellano, p134]

*377 **c** Endogenous peroxidase was not blocked; if the tissue contains many red blood cells or leukocytes blocking is essential. [Carson & Cappellano, pp274-286]

*378 **c** The mycoses are descriptive of diseases caused by fungi. [Carson & Cappellano, p215]

*379 **b** Myelin contains phospholipids in addition to protein, cholesterol, and cerebrosides. [Carson & Cappellano, p191]

*380 **c** In the Feulgen procedure, purines and pyrimidines are split from the sugar-phosphate grouping of DNA by hydrolysis. [Carson & Cappellano, p126]

*381 **a** The Churukian microwave modification of the Warthin-Starry technique will demonstrate cat-scratch disease (*Alipia felis*). [Carson & Cappellano, p236]

*382 **c** Rickettsiae are bacteria that do not possess the typical bacterial attributes. [Carson & Cappellano, p214]

*383 **d** The Grimelius procedure is suitable for demonstrating secretory granules in a carcinoid tumor as it will demonstrate both argyrophil and argentaffin granules. [Carson & Cappellano, pp251-253]

*384 **d** Cell blocks on cytology specimens make it easier to do special stains if needed because smears often require adaptations of the staining protocols and different controls. They are easy to prepare and frequently add diagnostic information. [Carson & Cappellano, p324]

*385 **c** The primary cells belonging to the lymphoreticular (immune) system are found in the thymus, lymph nodes, spleen, and bone marrow. [Young & Lowe, p208]

*386 **b** The enzyme involved in the technique shown (ATPase) belongs in the hydrolase class. [Carson & Cappellano, p297]

*387 **d** Chromaffin can be demonstrated by the Schmorl technique. [Bancroft & Gamble, p248]

*388 **d** Chromaffin-cell tumors of the adrenal gland are known as pheochromocytomas. [Carson & Cappellano, p7]

*389 **c**   Eosin Y rinses out of the cells faster than light green; therefore, rinsing for too long will produce false blue-green cells. [Carson & Cappellano, p327]

*390 **d**   Large type grouping is indicative of a neuropathic disease process. [Carson & Cappellano, p305]

*391 **c**   The final reaction product in the NADH diaphorase stain shown is a formazan. [Carson & Cappellano, p308]

*392 **c**   Antigen controls are not used; positive and negative controls are run with every antibody, and absorption controls are recommended in the characterization and evaluation of new antibodies. [Bancroft & Gamble, p453]

*393 **b**   The NADH diaphorase technique shown depends on the use of unfixed frozen sections. [Carson & Cappellano, pp308-309]

*394 **c**   The composition of the retrieval solution is very important in heat-induced epitope retrieval; the pH of the solution may vary between pH 3 and 9, metallic co-factors are involved in some enzyme reactions, and enzyme solution are used in enzyme-induced retrieval. [Carson & Cappellano, p266]

*395 **d**   The time should be increased in the lower dilution of dehydrating alcohols. The best eosin differentiation occurs in 70% alcohol. [Brown, p39]

*396 **a**   Tissue antigens are "stained" by fluorochrome labeled antibodies. [Carson & Cappellano, p269]

*397 **c**   Orcein can be used to demonstrate hepatitis B surface antigen. [Bancroft & Gamble, p325]

*398 **d**   Astrocytes are found predominately in the central nervous system. [Young & Lowe, pp140, 141]

*399 **a**   The slide is over impregnated and the technician should be asked to shorten the impregnation time in the future. Sections are bleached only if there is doubt about the stained material being melanin. [Carson & Cappellano, pppp248-250]

*400 **b**   A synapse is the contact between an axon of one neuron and the dendrite of another neuron. [Young & Lowe, pp122, 132]

*401 **d**   *Listeria monocytogenes* are tiny intracellular rods arranged in a "Chinese letter" formation and they stain variably with the Gram stain. [Bancroft & Gamble, p319]

*402 **d**   The problem of faint red staining of the muscle and muddy blue staining of the collagen is most likely the result of using old or depleted reagents. [Carson & Cappellano, p164]

*403 **d**   Lipofuscins may be demonstrated with a modified Ziehl-Neelsen carbol fuchsin technique using heat and prolonged staining. [Bancroft & Gamble, pp246-247]

*404 **b**   Colloidal gold can be used in both direct and indirect methods of immunostaining and has found wide usage in ultrastructural immunolocalization. [Bancroft & Gamble, p437]

*405 **b** Leucocyte common antibody (LCA) marks leucocytes, thus marking cells of lymphomas. [Carson & Cappellano, p277]

*406 **c** DAB (diaminobenzidine) was most likely the chromogen used in the image shown. [Carson & Cappellano, p291]

*407 **d** *Helicobacter pylori* are organisms found on gastric mucosa and are the presumptive cause of gastritis. [Bancroft & Gamble, p319]

*408 **c** The viability of Schiff reagent can be determined by adding a few drops of Schiff reagent to 10 mL of 37-40% formaldehyde. [Carson & Cappellano, p139]

*409 **a** A toluidine blue wet film is a good procedure for determining cellularity. [Carson & Cappellano, pp363-364]

*410 **b** There is an accumulation of copper in the liver in Wilson disease and the copper can be demonstrated by rubeanic acid. [Bancroft & Gamble, p250; Carson & Cappellano, p258]

*411 **c** Fungal cell walls contain carbohydrates which are oxidized to aldehydes; the aldehydes then react with Schiff reagent and give a positive PAS reaction. [Carson & Cappellano, p230]

*412 **a** Polyclonal antibodies bind to more than one epitope and their use may result in some nonspecific staining and crossreactivity. [Carson & Cappellano, p264; Kiernan, p489]

*413 **c** Only nuclei and Nissl substance should stain with cresyl echt violet in the LFB-CEV method. [Carson & Cappellano, pp207-208]

*414 **c** Of the antibodies listed, sarcomas will react positively with only vimentin. [Carson & Cappellano, p277]

*415 **c** Candidiasis is a very widespread and common fungal infection in man. [Bancroft & Gamble, p322]

*416 **a** The very dark staining fibers are Type I. [Carson & Cappellano, p305]

*417 **d** Nervous tissue is closely associated with Schwann cells in the peripheral nervous system and glial cells in the central nervous system. [Young & Lowe, pp127, 140]

*418 **c** Liver cytoplasm should not show any blue staining as it contains only scattered free ribosomes; if it does show basophilia, it is most likely that the hematoxylin was underdifferentiated. [Carson & Cappellano, p105; Young & Lowe, p290]

*419 **c** Auxochromes are ionizing groups that give the dye affinity for the tissue. [Carson & Cappellano, p110]

*420 **b** The nuclear bubbling is due to incomplete fixation. [Brown, pp8-9; Carson & Cappellano, pp26-28]

*421 **d** Chromaffin is normally found in the cells of the adrenal medulla as dark brown, granular material. [Bancroft & Gamble, p341]

*422 **c** The refractive index of the resinous mounting media used for sections should be ~1.53 - 1.54, which is the average refractive index of tissue; this gives the most transparency. [Carson & Cappellano, p132]

*423 **d** Formaldehyde is the reducing agent used in the Bielschowsky method. [Carson & Cappellano, pp196-197]

*424 **a** *Treponema pallidum* is a spirochete and will not stain with carbol-fuchsin solution. [Carson & Cappellano, p214]

*425 **a** The $-NH_2$ group is the most common basic auxochrome group encountered in dye chemistry. [Carson & Cappellano, p110]

*426 **b** Nissl substance is composed of large aggregates of granular endoplasmic reticulum with the RNA content providing the basis for demonstration by light microscopic techniques. Because of the RNA content, it can be demonstrated before and after extraction with ribonuclease. [Carson & Cappellano, p190; Kiernan, p228]

*427 **a** A common acidic auxochrome is $-COOH$; this is the acidic auxochrome of eosin. [Carson & Cappellano, p110]

*428 **b** A rhabdomyosarcoma is a malignant neoplasm of skeletal muscle. [Carson & Cappellano, ppxvi, 179]

*429 **b** The fungal organisms stained by the Grocott methenamine silver technique have been over impregnated. No internal structure can be seen in the organisms. [Carson & Cappellano, pp231-232]

*430 **d** Phosphorylases belong to the enzyme classification of transferases. [Carson & Cappellano, p298]

*431 **c** *Cryptococcus neoformans* can be differentially stained by Mayer mucicarmine; the other organisms will not stain with this method. [Bancroft & Gamble, p323; Carson & Cappellano, pp146, 215]

*432 **b** Copper can be demonstrated with hematoxylin without a mordant. [Bancroft & Gamble, p250; Kiernan, p351]

*433 **d** Type grouping, indicative of a neuropathy, is seen in the NADH diaphorase stain. [Carson & Cappellano, pp305]

*434 **a** ATPase stains normally fade over time. [Carson & Cappellano, p305]

*435 **d** Protease is used for some enzyme induced retrieval methods. [Carson & Cappellano, p269]

*436 **b** The von Kossa technique is the method of choice for demonstrating calcium phosphate in tissues. [Carson & Cappellano, p256]

*437 **c** The avidin-biotin complex (ABC) combines to the biotinylated secondary antibody. [Carson & Cappellano, p271]

*438 **c** The collagen is orange instead of red, indicating that the picric acid solution used in the preparation of van Gieson stain was not saturated. [Carson & Cappellano, p166]

*439 **d** One explanation for no immunostaining of either the patient or the positive control tissue is that either no primary antibody, or the wrong antibody was applied. [Carson & Cappellano, p286]

*440 **a** DAB provides a permanent preparation as sections using this chromogen can be mounted with a resinous mounting medium. They have a greater clarity, and the reaction product can be intensified if desired. [Carson & Cappellano, p269]

*441 **a** *Giardia duodenalis (lamblia)* can be demonstrated with the Giemsa stain. [Bancroft & Gamble, p329]

ISBN 978-089189-6494 ©ASCP 2016

*442 **d** The NADH diaphorase enzyme belongs to the oxidoreductase class. [Carson & Cappellano, p298]

*443 **c** *Borrelia burgdorferi* is the spirochete organism that causes Lyme disease and it can be demonstrated with the Steiner procedure. [Brown, p77; Carson & Cappellano, p214]

*444 **d** The origin of a malignant neoplasm positive for leukocyte common antigen and negative for carcinoembryonic antigen and cytokeratin is most likely the lymphatic system. [Carson & Cappellano, p277]

*445 **c** The PAP staining technique offers increased sensitivity of antigen detection over the direct or indirect conjugate methods. [Bancroft & Gamble, pp438-440; Carson & Cappellano, p271]

*446 **d** Some alcianophilic structures hydrate slowly, and will fail to stain intensely with alcian blue if not hydrated sufficiently. [Brown, p130]

*447 **d** Excessive asbestos exposure can lead to a tumor known as a mesothelioma. [Carson & Cappellano, p242]

*448 **c** The traditional direct technique, in which the antibody is commonly labeled with fluorescein isothiocyanate (FITC) or other fluorescent dyes for fluorescence microscopy is mainly confined to the demonstration of immunoglobulin and complement in frozen sections of skin and renal biopsies. [Bancroft & Gamble, p524]

*449 **b** The tissue is skeletal muscle. [Carson & Cappellano, pp294, 305]

*450 **c** A 60°C oven is not used for heat induced antigen retrieval. [Bancroft & Gamble, pp443-445; Carson & Cappellano, p282]

*451 **c** Actin and myosin form the thick and thin filaments of skeletal muscle fibers. [Young & Lowe, p107]

*452 **d** Alizarin red S forms a birefringent reaction product following staining of calcium deposits. [Carson & Cappellano, pp257-258]

*453 **a** The optimum hydrolysis time is fixative dependent, so a change in fixative would most likely indicate the need to change the time in 1 N HCl for the Feulgen stain. [Carson & Cappellano, pp126-127]

*454 **b** Enzymatically released naphthols, when coupled with diazonium salts, form an azo dye. [Carson & Cappellano, p301]

*455 **a** Alzheimer disease is characterized by neurofibrillary tangles, and deposits of amyloid surrounded radially by dilated and distorted neuronal processes to form senile plaques. [Bancroft & Gamble, p388; Carson & Cappellano, p196]

*456 **a** Validation of a new antibody does not involved the use of multiple chromogens; the chromogen normally used is the only one needed. [Carson & Cappellano, p273]

*457 **c** If the light green is not acidified, the appropriate charge on the cell cytoplasm will not be obtained and there will be no affinity for the counterstain. [Carson & Cappellano, pp109-110, 230]

Answers–Staining

Answers—Staining

*458 **b** Clean alcohol rinses after the counterstains are essential for optimal cytoplasmic staining; if the counterstain colors look "dirty," it is probably because of overused alcohol rinses. [Carson & Cappellano, p327]

*459 **a** Motor endplates can be demonstrated with the α-naphthyl acetate esterase stain. [Carson & Cappellano, p302]

*460 **d** When an ABC or streptavidin-biotin complex detection system is used, the likelihood of false positive staining in specific tissue types, such as liver and kidney, is high. [Carson & Cappellano, p285]

*461 **b** In Alzheimer disease, amyloid is deposited in the cortex and is surrounded radially by dilated and distorted neuronal process to form senile plaques. [Bancroft & Gamble, p388; Carson & Cappellano, pp200-201]

*462 **c** The periodic acid-Schiff stain can be used to demonstrate basement membranes. [Carson & Cappellano, pp139-141]

*463 **c** The Feulgen reaction utilized Schiff reagent. [Carson & Cappellano, p123]

*464 **a** HMB-45 is associated with the demonstration of melanin. [Carson & Cappellano, pp277-278]

*465 **b** The Holzer stain will stain glial fibers blue to purple. [Carson & Cappellano, p202-203]

*466 **d** Mycobacteria stain positive with the Truant auramine-rhodamine fluorescence technique. [Carson & Cappellano, pp221-222]

*467 **c** The activity of a nonspecific esterase enzyme is shown by an enzyme histochemical procedure. [Carson & Cappellano, p301]

*468 **d** The tissue shown is skin, with keratinizing stratified squamous epithelium seen; the other organs do not have keratinizing epithelium. [Young & Lowe, pp168, 169]

*469 **b** The collagen should stain a definite shade of pink, and should not have a grayish tone. [Brown, p37]

*470 **b** Acidophilic substances will bind eosin, basophilic substances will bind hematoxylin and sudanophilic components will bind any of the Sudan dyes. [Carson & Cappellano, pp110, 184]

*471 **c** In the alkaline phosphatase stain, the naphthol is coupled with diazonium. [Carson & Cappellano, p307]

*472 **d** The stain shown is the PTAH and it is not useful for the demonstration of pheochromocytomas. [Carson & Cappellano, pp178-179, 201]

*473 **c** The Grocott methenamine silver stain is best for the demonstration of *Pneumocystis jirovecii*. [Carson & Cappellano, p232]

*474 **a** An ideal Grocott fungal stain will show crisp black cell walls with a visible internal structure. [Carson & Cappellano, pp230-231]

*475 **d** The PAS stains neutral mucopolysaccharides, and the alcian blue and colloidal iron procedures stain acid mucopolysaccharides. [Carson & Cappellano, p138]

*476 **c** From one Z-line to the next in striated muscle is known as a sarcomere. [Young & Lowe, pp106, 107]

*477 **a** Acetic acid is added to Harris hematoxylin to improve selectivity of the stain for chromatin. [Carson & Cappellano, p113]

*478 **a** The Schmorl technique depends upon the reduction of ferric iron to ferrous iron, and the immediate binding to ferricyanide to give ferrous ferricyanide (Turnbull blue). [Carson & Cappellano, pp246-247]

*479 **b** Best carmine is a stain for glycogen and liver provides a good control. [Carson & Cappellano, pp143-144]

*480 **c** Bilirubin is oxidized to biliverdin (emerald green) by Fouchet reagent. [Carson & Cappellano, p255]

*481 **c** The tissue should be fixed for staining with HMB-45 antibody, one of the antibodies of choice for the demonstration of melanomas. [Carson & Cappellano, pp277-278]

*482 **d** The blue staining of myelin is due to the use of Luxol fast blue, a sulfonated copper phthalocyanine dye. [Carson & Cappellano, p206; Kiernan, p138]

*483 **b** The staining solution should have contained ferric chloride and potassium ferricyanide. [Carson & Cappellano, p247]

*484 **a** Problems with nuclear staining, especially the lack of sharply stained chromatin, is most often due to incomplete fixation. [Brown, p38; Carson & Cappellano, pp26, 125]

*485 **b** Optimum hydrolysis time should be determined for each fixative, but rarely does it exceed 15 minutes. Excessive hydrolysis will cause the lack of DNA demonstration. [Carson & Cappellano, p127]

*486 **b** The appropriate secondary antibody for a mouse primary would be an anti-mouse antibody, thus goat anti-mouse would be the choice of those listed. [Carson & Cappellano, p287]

*487 **d** The tunica adventitia is the tough outer coat of most arteries and is composed primarily of collagen, thus it would stain orange-red like collagen. [Young & Lowe, p152]

*488 **d** Gram positive organisms most likely will not stain correctly if the patient is taking antibiotics, because antibiotics compromise the cell walls. [Carson & Cappellano, p224]

*489 **c** The Sudan dyes are soluble in the fat. [Carson & Cappellano, p184]

*490 **b** The amino acid is positively charged and would attract the negatively charged eosin dye. [Carson & Cappellano, p110]

*491 **c** Robotic stainers permit different times in each compartment or container, but linear stainers require the same time for each container. With linear stainers, the differences in time needed for a solution can only be changed by changing the number of containers of a given solution. [Carson & Cappellano, p69]

*492 **c** The NADH diaphorase stain will demonstrate sarcoplasmic reticulum, Z-band material and mitochondria. [Carson & Cappellano, p308]

*493 **a** The majority of monoclonal antibodies are made in mice, so the secondary antibody would need to be an anti-mouse antibody. [Carson & Cappellano, p265]

*494 **b** Ribonucleic acid can be demonstrated by staining with pyronin. [Carson & Cappellano, pp127-129]

*495 **c** The auxochrome is the chemical group present in dyes that is responsible for forming ionic bonds. The amino and carboxyl groups are frequently occurring auxochromes. [Carson & Cappellano, p110]

*496 **c** Simultaneous coupling is a technique used in enzyme histochemistry. [Carson & Cappellano, p297]

*497 **d** The Color Index refers to a unique code, or identification, number that is used to reduce confusion. [Bancroft & Gamble, p116; Kiernan, p86]

*498 **d** Adsorption is a phenomenon influenced by the affinity of oppositely charged ions for each other. [Carson & Cappellano, p109]

*499 **c** The mucicarmine stain shown stains both sulfated and carboxylated mucin. [Carson & Cappellano, p144]

*500 **c** The naphthol AS-D chloroacetate esterase stain is useful in identifying granulocytes and mast cells; it is one of the rare enzyme techniques that will work on paraffin sections. [Carson & Cappellano, pp302-303]

*501 **b** A negative result on a Carnoy fixed control section of kidney known to contain amyloid is indicative of a staining or microtomy problem; Carnoy is the preferred fixation for Congo red staining. [Carson & Cappellano, p154]

*502 **c** Acidified pure methyl green is considered a specific stain for DNA. [Carson & Cappellano, p128]

*503 **c** Because the fibers are myelinated, the Weil stain will demonstrate the optic nerve. [Carson & Cappellano, pp204-205; Young & Lowe, p406]

*504 **c** A false negative acid-fast stain will most likely result if the tissue is fixed in Carnoy solution. [Carson & Cappellano, pp216-217]

*505 **b** Absorption occurs when tissue is penetrated by a dye solution and becomes colored without any other change or chemical reaction occurring. [Carson & Cappellano, p109]

*506 **b** The disruption of the tissue was most likely cause by excessively vigorous epitope retrieval. [Carson & Cappellano, p268]

*507 **a** A bottle of dye certified by the Biological Stain Commission shows the percentage by weight of the dye in the material; titration is only one test used in the certification process. [Kiernan, p88]

*508 **d** The pH of the eosin should be checked; the solution must be acidified in order to develop the appropriate charges for dye uptake by the cytoplasm. [Carson & Cappellano, pp109-110]

*509 **b** The tissue shown is a segment of the wall of the aorta. [Carson & Cappellano, p168; Young & Lowe, p157]

*510 **a** If the alcian blue staining time is prolonged, the nuclei will stain. [Brown, p129]

*511 **d** The most common cell of origin of insulinomas is the β cell of the pancreas. [Bancroft & Gamble, p284; Young & Lowe, p342]

Laboratory Operations

The following items have been identified as appropriate for both entry level histotechnicians and histotechnologists.

1   Which of the following protective equipment must be worn (by law) when one is handling formaldehyde?

    a impervious apron
    b lab coat
    c scrub suit
    d white uniform

2   The short-term exposure limit (STEL) for formaldehyde set by the Formaldehyde Standard is:

    a 0.5 ppm
    b 0.75 ppm
    c 1.0 ppm
    d 2.0 ppm

3   Which of the following may be disposed of in the sanitary sewer system according to Environmental Protection Agency (EPA) and Centers for Disease Control (CDC) guidelines?

    a absolute alcohol
    b silver salts
    c pulverized tissue
    d blood

4   500 mL of a 0.55% solution of potassium metabisulfite must be prepared. How many grams of potassium metabisulfite should be used?

    a 1.10
    b 2.75
    c 5.50
    d 11.0

5   Which of the following hazard classifications is of primary concern with picric acid?

    a mechanical
    b biologic
    c chemical
    d fire/explosion

6   The Formaldehyde Standard sets the time-weighted average (TWA) for formaldehyde at:

    a 0.5 ppm
    b 0.75 ppm
    c 1.0 ppm
    d 2.0 ppm

7   A temperature of 4°C is commonly associated with the laboratory:

    a flotation bath
    b incubator
    c refrigerator
    d freezer

8   Potassium dichromate falls into which of the following hazard classifications?

    a mechanical
    b biologic
    c chemical
    d fire/explosion

9   Which of the following pHs is considered basic?

    a 6.0
    b 6.5
    c 7.0
    d 7.5

10   A microscope with 2 eyepieces is:

    a monocular
    b binocular
    c achromatic
    d parfocal

11   When used in a National Fire Protection Association (NFPA) diamond, which of the following numbers is indicative of the most severe hazard?

    a 1
    b 2
    c 3
    d 4

12   Flammability hazards are indicated in which section of the NFPA diamond?

    a blue
    b red
    c yellow
    d white

13   According to the Environmental Protection Agency, it is illegal to dispose of concentrated acetic acid in the sanitary sewer system because it is classified as:

    a carcinogenic
    b corrosive
    c oxidizing
    d non-biodegradable

14   How many mL of water should be added to 80 mL of concentrated formaldehyde to obtain a solution of 10% formalin?

    a 360
    b 720
    c 800
    d 920

15   During microscopic examination, if the section remains in focus when changing objectives, the objectives are:

    a binocular
    b achromatic
    c apochromatic
    d parfocal

16   Paraffin sections of brain are cut at 15 micrometers. This is equivalent to how many millimeters?

    a 1.5
    b 0.15
    c 0.015
    d 0.0015

17   A 0.5% solution of light green is needed. The bottle contains only 4.25 grams of dye powder. How many mL of solution can be prepared if all of the dye is used?

    a 212
    b 425
    c 850
    d 1700

18   The handling of biohazards is governed by the:

    a Blood-borne Pathogen Standard
    b Formaldehyde Standard
    c Laboratory Standard
    d Respiratory Protection Standard

19   A solution is prepared that contains 5 g of NaCl in 200 mL of water. This is equivalent to which of the following percent solutions?

    a 0.4
    b 1.0
    c 2.5
    d 5.0

20   Acid-fast bacilli may be demonstrated by staining with auromine-rhodamine and then examined with this type of microscope:

    a electron
    b darkfield
    c fluorescence
    d light

21   The cause of Creutzfeldt-Jakob disease falls into which of the following categories:

    a viruses
    b fungi
    c prions
    d protozoans

22   Ethyl alcohol may be disposed of in the sewer system if it:

    a was not used on the tissue processor
    b contains methanol to make it unfit for drinking
    c is less than 24% alcohol
    d has never been treated in a solvent recycler

23   To obtain a total magnification of 1000 with an ocular of 10× magnification, the objective must have a magnification of:

    a 10×
    b 100×
    c 450×
    d 1000×

24   Fires involving wood and paper are considered:

    a Class A fires
    b Class B fires
    c Class C fires
    d Class D fires

25 During microscopic review of H&E stained sections, it is noted that there is insufficient light on the slide. The BEST way to correct this is by:

  a changing to a higher objective
  b increasing the numerical aperture
  c lowering the substage condenser
  d opening the iris diaphragm

26 Organic solvents should be disposed of by:

  a pouring them down a sink and flushing with plenty of water
  b collecting them in waste containers for future disposal or distillation
  c pouring them into a deep pit in the ground
  d collecting them in old bottles and storing in a vacant building

27 500 mL of 3% alcian blue in 1% acetic acid contains:

  a 1 g alcian blue, 3 mL acetic acid, and 497 mL water
  b 3 g alcian blue, 1 mL acetic acid, and 499 mL water
  c 15 g alcian blue, 5 mL acetic acid, and 495 mL water
  d 15 g alcian blue, 1 mL acetic acid, and 499 mL water

28 Another way of expressing 350 mg is:

  a 3.50 g
  b 0.35 g
  c 0.035 g
  d 0.0035 g

29 Following staining with a solution prepared from a new bottle of eosin dye powder, the color results are not the same as those obtained with the previously used eosin dye powder. The BEST course of action is to:

  a discard the new dye and reorder
  b use an eosin substitute
  c try another formula for the new eosin
  d determine whether both dyes have the same dye content

30 Components of living tissue do NOT require staining if they are to be examined by:

  a fluorescent microscopy
  b light microscopy
  c phase contrast microscopy
  d transmission electron microscopy

31 An acidic or alkaline substance added to a solution to prevent a change in pH is called a(n):

  a differentiator
  b oxidizer
  c catalyst
  d buffer

32   The "high dry" objective usually has a magnification of:

   a 4×
   b 10×
   c 20×
   d 45×

33   A section 5 micrometers thick would be equivalent to how many millimeters in thickness?

   a 0.0005
   b 0.005
   c 0.05
   d 0.5

34   Which of the following documents must be available to all laboratory employees according to the Hazard Communication Standard?

   a First Responder Incident reports
   b Biohazard Disposal instructions for the gross room
   c Material Safety Data Sheet on chemicals in laboratory
   d Formaldehyde Exposure reduction plan

35   How much 95% alcohol must be used to prepare 1000 mL of 70% alcohol?

   a 271 mL
   b 316 mL
   c 714 mL
   d 737 mL

36   Flammable liquids should always be stored:

   a in flammable storage cabinets
   b in glass containers
   c in a separate building from the laboratory
   d above eye level

37   To prepare 50 mL of 2% ferric chloride from a 10% solution, how many mL of the 10% solution will be required?

   a 5
   b 10
   c 20
   d 25

38   Doubly refractile particles are also called:

   a isotropic
   b fluorescent
   c birefringent
   d reflective

39 The microwave oven can be used to fix tissue because of the:

    a rapid molecular movement
    b reaction between protein molecules
    c ionizing radiation
    d rupture of hydrogen bonds

40 How many mL of water should be added to 100 mL of a 20% solution of silver nitrate to obtain a 10% solution?

    a 20
    b 50
    c 100
    d 200

41 To prepare 500 mL of 0.55% potassium metabisulfite solution, how many grams of potassium metabisulfite would be required?

    a 1.10
    b 2.75
    c 5.50
    d 11.0

42 A reagent labeled with a NFPA diamond has a 4 in the blue quadrant. This means that:

    a there is no hazard
    b there is a slight hazard
    c the material may be harmful if inhaled or absorbed
    d the hazard is extreme and exposure could result in death

43 Before adjusting the pH of the Warthin-Starry staining solution, the pH meter should be calibrated with a buffer solution of pH:

    a 4.0
    b 6.0
    c 7.0
    d 10.0

44 One cubic centimeter is equal to:

    a 0.01 liter
    b 0.1 liter
    c 1 milliliter
    d 10 milliliters

45   The number 4 placed in the red quadrant of the National Fire Protection Association (NFPA) diamond shown below would indicate a chemical that:

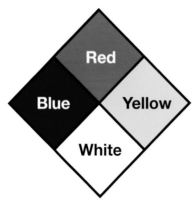

    a can cause death on short exposure
    b is very reactive and may detonate
    c can be easily ignited at room temperature
    d is a very strong oxidizer

46   Some striated muscle cells are as much as 400 millimeters in length. This is equivalent to how many centimeters?

    a 0.04
    b 0.4
    c 4.0
    d 40

47   The ability of a microscope objective to separate small detail is the:

    a numerical aperture
    b depth of focus
    c virtual image
    d resolving power

48   A fire involving hydrocarbon reagents is classified as a:

    a Class A fire
    b Class B fire
    c Class C fire
    d Class D fire

49   One gallon of a laboratory solvent has spilled on the laboratory floor. What is the approximate square footage (sq ft) of space the spill will cover?

    a 1 sq ft
    b 10 sq ft
    c 20 sq ft
    d 30 sq ft

50 According to the Environmental Protection Agency (EPA), the ONLY disposal method approved for pathologic waste is:

    a by sterilization
    b in a sharps container
    c by incineration
    d in a local landfill

51 When using micrometer pipettes for measuring liquids, it is recommended that:

    a pipettes should be stored in a drawer along with the tips
    b the same pipette be used for volumes of 0.5 to 1000 μL
    c calibration of pipettes be checked annually
    d pipettes should be held at 45° angle for best accuracy of the draw

52 A temperature of 37°C is most commonly associated with:

    a the flotation bath
    b the laboratory incubator
    c paraffin infiltration
    d room temperature

53 Robotic type automated slide stainers are considered:

    a inflexible for use with various staining protocols
    b unsafe because of solvent fumes exhausted into the lab
    c to allow exact staining times in any given station
    d to require excess technical personnel time

54 How many mL of 29% ferric chloride stock solution should be used when preparing 50 mL of 2% ferric chloride?

    a 1.16
    b 3.45
    c 6.90
    d 7.25

55 Which of the following is the formula for calculating a percent (w/v) solution?

    a (grams of solute × 100)/(volume of solvent)
    b (grams of solute) × (volume of solvent) × (100)
    c (volume of solvent × 100)/(grams of solute)
    d (grams of solute) × (volume of solvent)/(100)

56 How many mL of 10% sodium hydroxide are required to prepare 200 mL of a 4% solution?

    a 8
    b 20
    c 40
    d 80

57   The symbol below posted in an area would indicate which of the following hazards?

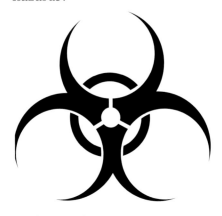

   a electrical
   b radiation
   c biohazard
   d explosive

58   Solvent recovery systems are able to separate contaminants from solvents because the contaminants:

   a are acids and the solvents are bases
   b differ in boiling points from the solvents
   c differ in solubility from the solvents
   d are larger molecules than the solvents

59   During a microwave Grocott staining procedure, the methenamine silver reagent boils. In response to this, one should:

   a not be concerned; this is an expected event
   b decrease the heating time of the reagent
   c use a larger container for the reagent
   d switch to a different staining procedure

60   The type of microtome used for routine paraffin block sectioning is:

   a sliding
   b vibrating
   c rotary
   d ultramicrotome

61   What volume of a stock solution of 25% NaCl would be required to prepare 250 mL of a 5% solution?

   a 5 mL
   b 12.5 mL
   c 25 mL
   d 50 mL

62 To help prevent repetitive motion injury or other musculoskeletal disorder, it is recommended that technicians:

    a rock the microtome handwheel with wrist extension and flexion
    b keep microtomy tools at a workspace away from the microtome in use
    c rest forearms and wrists on the sharp edges of work surfaces
    d take short "stretch" breaks from repetitive tasks every 20-30 minutes

63 Polarizing microscopes use a polarizer and a(n):

    a barrier filter
    b diffuser
    c analyzer
    d refractometer

64 A researcher asks that sections of tissue be cut at 70 micrometers. This is equivalent to how many millimeters in thickness?

    a 0.0007
    b 0.007
    c 0.07
    d 0.7

65 A solution contains 20 g of solute dissolved in 0.5 L of water. What is the percentage of this solution?

    a 2%
    b 4%
    c 10%
    d 20%

66 How many milliliters of a 3% solution can be made if 6 grams of solute are used?

    a 100 mL
    b 200 mL
    c 400 mL
    d 600 mL

67   When the symbol below is posted, material stored in the area requires:

    a shielding or containment techniques
    b that employees wear personal protective equipment around it
    c storage in a biologic safety cabinet
    d protection from an ignition source

68   When a solution containing hydrochloric acid is to be discarded in the sink, it should be:

    a neutralized to pH 7.0
    b between pH 3 and pH 11
    c diluted to less than 24%
    d followed by an alkaline solution

69   A small electrical fire occurs in the laboratory. Which of the following substances would be appropriate for use in extinguishing the fire?

    a water
    b soda acid
    c carbon tetrachloride
    d carbon dioxide

70   When immersion oil has been used for microscopic review of microorganisms in a tissue section, it is important to remove the oil from the objective lens immediately:

    a with xylene-soaked gauze
    b with lens paper
    c by removing the objective and washing it in water
    d by wiping it with a paper towel

71   Plastic or glass containers should be used in a microwave oven because:

    a they are microwave transparent
    b they have the same properties as metal containers
    c liquids heat evenly in glass and plastic containers
    d liquids do not generate fumes when heated in plastic or glass

72   One micron is equal to:

   a 0.001 meters
   b 0.0001 meters
   c 0.00001 meters
   d 0.000001 meters

73   A chemical that should be used under a hood because of the possibility of extreme respiratory irritation is:

   a picric acid
   b diaminobenzidine
   c hydrochloric acid
   d chromic acid

74   The major benefit of using a microwave oven in the histology laboratory is that:

   a the space required for the instrument is small
   b procedures performed using the microwave oven take less time
   c liquids heat uniformly in the microwave oven
   d inexpensive, household microwave ovens are recommended

75   How many grams of aniline blue should be used to prepare 750 mL of a 5% solution?

   a 3.8
   b 37.5
   c 50.0
   d 75.0

76   To increase paraffin embedded tissue section adherence to the slide, it is recommended to:

   a use heated slides
   b cut all sections at 6 μm thickness
   c pick up sections onto charged or plus slides
   d decalcify bone sections only in EDTA

77   An employee complains of tingling or numbness in the hands, an aching neck, and shoulder and wrist pain. Referral to the health clinic would most likely reveal that the employee has:

   a bursitis
   b carpal tunnel syndrome
   c chronic repetitive trauma
   d range of motion inadequacy

78 The laboratory supervisor is talking about a new LIS. She is referring to which of the following:

   a Laboratory Instrumentation System
   b Laboratory Information Standards
   c Laboratory Information System
   d Laboratory Instrumentation Standards

79 The type of microscope used to capture the image seen here is:

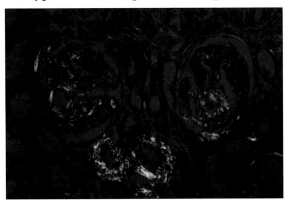

   a fluorescence
   b polarizing
   c light
   d electron

80 The function of the condenser on the light microscope is to:

   a concentrate light on the tissue specimen
   b magnify and resolve the image
   c regulate the intensity of light illuminating the specimen
   d furnish strongly divergent light to the specimen

81 When the technician removes waste paraffin wax from the embedding center, by which of the following methods should the wax be disposed?

   a collected for a licensed waste hauler
   b drain disposal
   c in the trash
   d treat in solvent recovery equipment

82 The possibility of repetitive motion injury (RMI) may be reduced by:

   a using a rocking motion of the flywheel when cutting paraffin sections
   b tightly gripping the forceps when embedding and coverslipping
   c removing the lid of each cassette with the left thumb
   d utilizing an automated coverslipping system

83 After completion of a reticulin staining procedure, the technician must dispose of the waste uranyl nitrate. What is the appropriate method for its disposal?

    a drain disposal without any treatment
    b incineration
    c collection for waste hauler pick-up
    d combine with sulfuric acid for inactivation, then drain disposal

The following items (*) have been identified as more appropriate for entry level histotechnologists.

*84 100 mL of a 1% solution of Luxol fast blue is needed. The old, stock dye had a dye concentration of 80% and the new preparation has a dye concentration of 84%. To achieve the same consistency in staining as with the old dye, how many grams of the new dye are required?

    a 0.95
    b 1.0
    c 1.05
    d 1.4

*85 An employee wears a lab coat while assisting in the gross dissection area. This employee is later seen in the cafeteria in the same lab coat, indicating that:

    a the employee needs further training
    b lab coats should not be used in the gross dissection area
    c only street clothes should be worn to the cafeteria
    d the employee is conforming with a perfectly acceptable practice

*86 How many grams of solute are required to prepare 500 mL of a 0.2 N solution of $CaCl_2$ (atomic weights are Ca = 40.08, Cl = 35.45)?

    a 2.22
    b 5.55
    c 11.1
    d 22.2

*87 1 mL of a 1:50 dilution of antibody is needed. How many microliters of the primary antibody would be needed?

    a 0.2
    b 2.0
    c 20.0
    d 200.0

*88 Which of the following solutions is considered hazardous and may NOT be disposed of in the sanitary sewer system?

   a silver nitrate
   b copper sulfate
   c zinc sulfate
   d ferric chloride

*89 The domain of learning that deals with levels of understanding knowledge is:

   a affective
   b motor development
   c synthesis
   d cognitive

*90 The cryostat used in the surgical suite has stopped cooling properly. To be in compliance with the Blood-borne Pathogen Standard, before having someone service the equipment, the cryostat should:

   a be decontaminated
   b be allowed to air dry
   c be cleaned of debris
   d have the microtome removed

*91 How many grams of Na_2SO_4 (atomic weights are Na = 23, S = 32, O = 16) are required to prepare 500 mL of a 2 M solution?

   a 35.5
   b 71.0
   c 142.0
   d 284.0

*92 500 mL of a 0.2% solution of light green is needed. The old, stock dye had a dye concentration of 90% and the new preparation has a dye concentration of 85%. To achieve the same consistency in staining as with the old dye, how many grams of the new dye are required?

   a 0.85
   b 0.94
   c 1.06
   d 1.88

*93 The educational process is enhanced if the teacher and learner both have a clear definition of the expected:

   a grade
   b learning outcomes
   c career
   d assessment methods

*94 A special staining procedure has been ordered on tissue from a patient suspected to have amyloidosis. What type of microscope is required for the mandatory secondary examination of the stained slide for diagnosis?

    a polarizing
    b light
    c electron
    d fluorescence

*95 100 µL (microliters) equals:

    a 0.1 mL
    b 0.01 mL
    c 0.001 mL
    d 0.0001 mL

*96 When writing cognitive level instructional objectives, some of the verbs which should be used in "recall" level objectives are:

    a interpret, compose, or design
    b define, describe, identify
    c calculate, operate, solve
    d differentiate, relate, modify

*97 Plastic resins require more specialized handling techniques than waxes because resins:

    a may cause dermatitis
    b require manual embedding
    c are used at high temperatures
    d harden instantly

*98 Which of the following completes the educational learning objective describing a student learning technical skills during a clinical rotation in the histopathology laboratory?

    "Upon completion of the clinical rotation, the student should be able to:
    a cut 20 slides within 30 minutes with less than 5 artifacts"
    b list the 3 parts of the embedding center"
    c define the steps of workflow in a histology laboratory"
    d describe 5 microtomy artifacts"

*99 How many grams of NaOH (MW = 40) are required to prepare 500 mL of a 0.25 M solution?

    a 5
    b 10
    c 12.5
    d 20

*100 The primary antibody must be diluted 1:100 for an immunohistochemical procedure. How many microliters of the primary antibody would be required to prepare a total volume of 2 mL?

  a 2
  b 10
  c 20
  d 100

*101 The agency which sets standards for and accredits laboratory education/ training programs is:

  a American Society for Clinical Pathology (ASCP)
  b Board of Certification (BOC)
  c National Accrediting Agency for Clinical Laboratory Sciences (NAACLS)
  d National Coalition for Allied Health Leadership (NCAHL)

*102 In order for the laboratory to be prepared for possible chemical spills, the following are organizing procedures EXCEPT for:

  a take an inventory of all chemicals in the laboratory
  b plan for small and large spills
  c decide on a plan for disposal of spill clean-up materials
  d determine a method for reduction of the use of hazardous chemicals

*103 The use of chloroform in the histology laboratory requires safety precautions because it is:

  a very reactive
  b flammable
  c a carcinogen
  d corrosive

*104 The recommended method for testing the amount of suction a hood exhaust system has is to:

  a hold a lens paper inside the hood to see if it is pulled by the suction
  b close all air conditioning vents near the hood and check for chemical fumes by smell
  c use a tracer gas or smoke for the initial evaluation
  d use ozone generators to validate the amount of suction

*105 The Equal Employment Opportunity (EEO) executive order which prohibits discrimination in employment decisions on the basis of race, color, religion, sex, or national origin, is also known as:

  a Affirmative Action
  b Civil Rights Act
  c Equal Pay Act
  d Americans with Disabilities Act

*106 As it relates to hiring practices, the Age Discrimination in Employment Act (ADEA) prohibits discrimination against any person of this age or older:

    a 30
    b 40
    c 50
    d 60

*107 A change in the pH of a solution from 7 to 6 indicates that the solution now contains:

    a double the number of hydronium ions as before
    b 5 times the number of hydronium ions as before
    c 10 times the number of hydronium ions as before
    d double the number of hydroxyl ions as before

*108 During an employment interview, which of the following inquiries CANNOT be asked of the interviewee?

    a tell me about your educational background
    b describe 2 things that motivate you at work
    c tell me about your family and children
    d what experiences led you to this career?

*109 Psychomotor objectives relate to teaching and learning:

    a knowledge and facts
    b technical skills
    c behaviors
    d dependability

*110 Which of the following agencies provide fire safety standards that must be followed in the laboratory?

    a ASCP & CAP
    b FDA & HCFA
    c OSHA & NFPA
    d NSH & AMA

*111 Side-by-side comparisons are a means of instrument:

    a verification
    b validation
    c certification
    d monitoring

*112 The Laboratory Accreditation Program of the College of American Pathologists (LAP-CAP) accredits:

   a only laboratories as required by CLIA
   b entire healthcare organizations as required by CLIA
   c entire healthcare organizations on a voluntary basis
   d only laboratories on a voluntary basis

*113 The phase of workflow that deals with interpretation and reporting of laboratory processes is:

   a preanalytical
   b analytical
   c postanalytical
   d LEAN

*114 After receipt of formaldehyde monitoring results, management must notify employees within how many days?

   a 15
   b 30
   c 45
   d 60

*115 A laboratory supervisor is administering an annual Competency-Based performance evaluation in microtomy to a histotechnician. What is the correct method for this type of evaluation to be done?

   a the histotechnician signs a form stating that he/she can perform the tasks being evaluated
   b the supervisor asks the histotechnician if he/she can perform the tasks being evaluated
   c the supervisor watches the technician to document that he/she is performing the task to established standards
   d the histotechnician assures the supervisor that he/she met the competency-based standards while no one else was in the lab

*116 The overtime budget for the laboratory is \$38,773, but \$50,419 has already been spent. What percent over budget does this represent?

   a 33%
   b 70%
   c 77%
   d 100%

*117 A one Normal solution is equivalent to:

   a 1 mole of solute per kilogram of solvent
   b 1 mole of solute per 100 mL of solution
   c 1 gram equivalent weight of solute per 1 L of solution
   d 2 moles of solute per 1 L of solution

ISBN 978-089189-6494 ©ASCP 2016

*118 Which of the following is the formula for calculating the gram equivalent weight of a chemical?

    a MW × valence
    b MW ÷ valence
    c MW + valence
    d MW – valence

*119 The proper microscope for examining tissue stained with thioflavin T is the:

    a electron
    b light
    c polarizing
    d fluorescence

*120 600 µL of antiserum are added to 2400 µL of diluent will give a final dilution of:

    a 1:5
    b 1:50
    c 1:500
    d 1:5000

*121 A document that lists the essential functions of a job, defined as those that are most important and/or performed most often, is known as the:

    a job posting
    b personnel action form
    c position description
    d performance review

*122 A laboratory has received its new H&E stainer. In order to assure that it will function consistently as expected, before it is put into routine use the laboratory must perform a:

    a waiver certificate from CLIA
    b variable cost analysis
    c visual examination of working parts
    d validation process

*123 A dangerous materials warning system chart developed by the NFPA is in use in the laboratory. A reagent is identified with a red background and the number three (3). This indicates a compound that:

    a will cause irritation if not treated
    b is unstable and may spontaneously explode
    c is flammable and will easily ignite
    d should be stored in an explosion proof cabinet

*124 To maximize the resolving power of a light microscope, the substage condenser should be adjusted to sharply focus the light on the:

   a condenser front lens
   b lamp filament
   c specimen slide
   d iris diaphragm

*125 The number of hours used to calculate the annual salary of a full time employee is:

   a 1920
   b 1950
   c 2080
   d 2800

*126 While using a 10× objective to view an H&E stained section, the section appears bright with well stained nuclei. When the objective is changed to 40×, the section appears dark and detail is obscured. This problem most likely could be corrected by:

   a restaining the section and decreasing the hematoxylin
   b slightly opening the iris diaphragm
   c using the 90× objective
   d cleaning the ocular

*127 Which of the following is the formula for calculating the molarity of a solution?

   a number of moles of solute per liter of solution
   b number of moles of solute × 100
   c 1 GEW of solute × 10
   d 1 GEW of solute per liter of solution

*128 How many mL of 85% alcohol is required to make 5000 mL of 60% alcohol?

   a 352.94
   b 2607.40
   c 3529.40
   d 3534.90

*129 When cognitive lesson objectives are well written, the intended learning outcomes should be clear to the learner and they should also:

   a be easy to measure through testing
   b contain no measurable outcomes
   c measure student behaviors such as dependability
   d measure microtomy skill quality

*130 Most histology laboratories have discontinued using a specific chemical because it is a severe skin irritant, corrosive to metals, is a severe environmental hazard and requires licensed waste hauler disposal. Which of the following chemicals has these characteristics?

a silver nitrate
b mercury
c zinc
d limonene

*131 The gross dissection area is being remodeled. Ventilation must be designed to ensure that the exposure to formaldehyde over an 8-hour period, or the time-weighted average (TWA), is no more than:

a 0.5 ppm
b 0.75 ppm
c 1.0 ppm
d 1.5 ppm

*132 The laboratory's supply of nitrile gloves has been depleted. One of the technicians develops an itchy rash on her hands after wearing the replacement latex gloves in the lab for prolonged periods each day for one week before the nitrile gloves are received. What is a probable cause of her discomfort?

a latex is a sensitizer and she has developed contact dermatitis
b the technician didn't wash the gloves after changing the processor
c after nitrile gloves are discontinued, it is common for a rash to appear
d nitrile gloves allow formaldehyde to penetrate, causing dermatitis that continued to worsen

*133 The time weighted average (TWA) of exposure to formaldehyde has been shown by monitoring to be 0.7 parts per million. According to OSHA regulations for the permissible exposure limit (PEL), the TWA must be:

a corrected within 15 days
b re-monitored within 15 days
c re-monitored within 6 months
d reported to the employee within 5 days

*134 Consider the learning objective:

"Upon completion of the clinical rotation in the histopathology laboratory, the student will exhibit dependability in attendance according to laboratory policy."

Into which category does this objective fit?

a affective
b didactic
c psychomotor
d cognitive

*135 The microscopist is examining an FITC stained section with a fluorescence microscope and thinks that there is some background autofluorescence. Of the following, which is most likely to autofluoresce?

a collagen fibers
b urate crystals
c talc or silica
d elastic fibers

*136 The numerical aperture of the objective lens:

a is unaffected by immersion media
b defines the expected resolving power of the microscope
c increases as the resolving power of the microscope decreases
d is greater with a high dry objective than with an oil immersion objective

*137 When a laboratory focuses on the process rather than on the end product or service by evaluating errors and addressing resolutions, that program is known as:

a risk monitoring
b quality assurance
c assessment surveys
d risk control

*138 Bloom's Taxonomy Levels refer to the:

a workbook used in clinical laboratory training
b cognitive domain with progression from beginner to expert in thought processes
c amount of work produced in a given amount of time
d program that assures employees are providing consistent and reliable results

*139 Which of the following inquiries can be legally made regarding a job applicant's affiliations?

a private organization affiliations
b specific jobs or social organizations that relate to the position the applicant is seeking
c religious affiliations of the applicant, including any holidays observed
d political affiliations

*140 The document which defines what is expected of an employee in a specific position is known as the:

a work schedule
b procedure manual
c job description
d job analysis

*141 A histology tissue processor costs $42,000, has a life expectancy of 6 years and a guaranteed trade-in value of $8,000, and will handle 9,000 specimens a year. Calculate its yearly depreciation allowance using straight-line depreciation.

  a $7,750
  b $5,666
  c $34,000
  d $3,777

*142 The Histology section of the laboratory had 12,652 labor hours for the year. How many FTEs were used by this section?

  a 4.4
  b 5.7
  c 6.1
  d 9.2

*143 Which of the following has been established to ensure that a person is minimally competent to enter the practice of histotechnology?

  a accreditation
  b certification
  c credentialing
  d licensure

*144 Consider this objective written for a lecture on fixation.

  "Following successful completion of this lecture, the student should be able to list 3 functions of a fixative."

  In which domain level does this objective belong?

  a psychomotor
  b cognitive
  c affective
  d evaluation

*145 HIPAA is concerned with which of the following :

  a infection control
  b formaldehyde standards
  c patient privacy
  d ergonomics

*146 Which part of laboratory safety operations is NOT covered by a federal regulation?

  a blood and surgical tissue handling
  b ergonomics while working
  c fire safety
  d formaldehyde labeling

*147 When a new undiluted antibody is received in the laboratory, which of the following procedures must be followed?

   a begin routine use on patient cases immediately
   b keep the new antibody frozen until the antibody currently in use is totally depleted
   c validation testing of various dilutions of the new antibody on known positive and negative tissue samples
   d use on patient tissue at the undiluted concentration

*148 A method used for evaluating psychomotor domain objectives is to have a student:

   a calculate the percentage of a working solution using a mathematical formula
   b list the steps of a staining procedure in correct order
   c perform microtomy without artifacts on various tissue blocks
   d demonstrate respectful communication with fellow students

*149 The quality management assessment process that is designed as an educational program to improve the preparation of histologic slides in laboratories nationwide is called:

   a ASCP Board of Certification examinations
   b NAACLS accreditation for training programs
   c CAP laboratory inspections
   d NSH/CAP HistoQIP challenges

*150 After completion of the staining procedure shown here, how should the technician dispose of the oxidizer used?

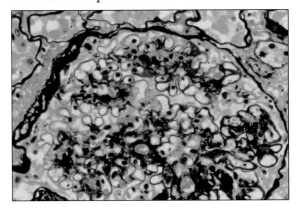

   a drain disposal without pretreatment
   b neutralization and then drain disposal
   c incineration
   d collect for licensed waste hauler

*151 Scanning a barcode at each workstation can assist the supervisor in all of the following EXCEPT in:

   a reducing human error
   b determining each employee's productivity
   c calculating reagents needed for staining
   d paperless procedure manuals

*152 The square object to the left of the surgical number on the cassette in this image is useful for all of the following EXCEPT:

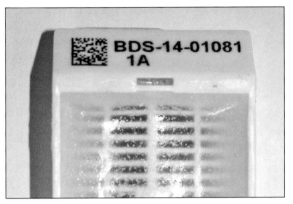

   a staining protocols
   b decreasing specimen mix-ups
   c determining employee productivity
   d real time specimen tracking

*153 Pictograms are required on labels under the:

   a Formaldehyde Standard
   b Bloodborne Pathogen Standard
   c Hazard Communication 2012
   d Ergonomics Standard

*154 Which of the following is required on chemical labels under the revised Hazard Communication Standard?

   a NFPA hazard label
   b signal words
   c disposal instructions
   d infection hazard

Answer Key–Laboratory Operations

The following items have been identified as appropriate for both entry level histotechnicians and histotechnologists.

1 a	15 d	29 d	43 a	57 c	71 a
2 d	16 c	30 c	44 c	58 b	72 d
3 d	17 c	31 d	45 c	59 b	73 c
4 b	18 a	32 d	46 d	60 c	74 b
5 d	19 c	33 b	47 d	61 d	75 b
6 b	20 c	34 c	48 b	62 d	76 c
7 c	21 c	35 d	49 c	63 c	77 c
8 c	22 c	36 a	50 c	64 c	78 c
9 d	23 b	37 b	51 c	65 b	79 b
10 b	24 a	38 c	52 b	66 b	80 a
11 d	25 d	39 a	53 c	67 d	81 c
12 b	26 b	40 c	54 b	68 b	82 d
13 b	27 c	41 b	55 a	69 d	83 c
14 b	28 b	42 d	56 d	70 b	

The following items (*) have been identified as more appropriate for entry level histotechnologists.

*84 a	*96 b	*108 c	*120 a	*132 a	*144 b
*85 a	*97 a	*109 b	*121 c	*133 c	*145 c
*86 b	*98 a	*110 c	*122 d	*134 a	*146 b
*87 c	*99 a	*111 b	*123 c	*135 a	*147 c
*88 a	*100 c	*112 d	*124 c	*136 b	*148 c
*89 d	*101 c	*113 c	*125 c	*137 b	*149 d
*90 a	*102 d	*114 a	*126 b	*138 b	*150 a
*91 c	*103 c	*115 c	*127 a	*139 b	*151 d
*92 c	*104 c	*116 a	*128 c	*140 c	*152 a
*93 b	*105 a	*117 c	*129 a	*141 b	*153 c
*94 a	*106 b	*118 b	*130 b	*142 c	*154 b
*95 a	*107 c	*119 d	*131 b	*143 b	

ISBN 978-089189-6494   ©ASCP 2016

The following items have been identified as appropriate for both entry level histotechnicians and histotechnologists.

1 **a** An apron or lab coat that is impervious to liquids is required as part of the Formaldehyde Standard. [Carson & Cappellano, p14]

2 **d** The Formaldehyde Standard sets the STEL at 2.0 ppm. [Carson & Cappellano, p14; Dapson, p22]

3 **d** Blood may be disposed in the sewer system according to the EPA and CDC guidelines. [Carson & Cappellano, p87]

4 **b** 2.75 grams of potassium metabisulfite is needed. Use the percentage formula (% desired :100 = g or mL needed : volume desired) for this calculation. [Carson & Cappellano, p98]

5 **d** Picric acid is explosive, especially when dry, shocked, heated, or in contact with metals or metallic salts. [Carson & Cappellano, p91]

6 **b** The Formaldehyde Standard sets the TWA at 0.75 ppm. [Carson & Cappellano, p89; Dapson, p22]

7 **c** The laboratory refrigerator should be maintained at a temperature of 4-10°C, so that the contents are not allowed to freeze nor to get too warm. [Carson & Cappellano, p78]

8 **c** Potassium dichromate is a chemical hazard classified as a toxin and a carcinogen, corrosive to eyes, skin and mucous membranes, and is a strong oxidizer. [Dapson, pp35, 266]

9 **d** A pH above 7 is considered basic or alkaline. [Carson & Cappellano, p78]

10 **b** The term "binocular" refers to having 2 eyepieces. [Carson & Cappellano, ppxii]

11 **d** The NFPA diamond uses numbers 1-4 to indicate severity of hazards, with 4 indicating the greatest hazard. [Carson & Cappellano, p94; Dapson, p125]

12 **b** The red portion of the NFPA diamond indicates flammability hazards. [Carson & Cappellano, p94]

13 **b** Corrosive liquids, such as acetic acid, cannot be put into the sewer system. [Carson & Cappellano, p93; Dapson, p136]

14 **b** Use the percentage formula (%desired :100 = g or mL needed :volume desired) for calculating the answer of 720 mL. [Carson & Cappellano, p98]

15 **d** The term "parfocal" indicates that the section will remain in focus even when changing objectives. [Carson & Cappellano, p54]

16 **c** 15 micrometers (μm) is equal to 0.015 mL. [Carson & Cappellano, p101]

17 **c** Use the percentage formula (%desired :100 = g or mL needed :volume desired) for calculating the answer of 850. [Carson & Cappellano, p98]

18 **a** The Blood-borne Pathogen Standard governs biohazard handling. [Carson & Cappellano, p86; Dapson, p53]

19 **c** Use the percentage formula (%desired :100 = g or mL needed :volume desired) for calculating the answer of 2.5%. [Carson & Cappellano, p98]

20 **c** The auramine-rhodamine procedure uses a fluorescent dye to demonstrate the acid-fast bacilli, and must be examined with a fluorescence microscope. [Carson & Cappellano, pp221-222]

21   **c**   Creutzfeldt-Jakob disease (CJD) is caused by a prion, which is an abnormal protein. The prions are resistant to many processes used in histology that normally kill other pathogens, and are only susceptible to autoclaving at high temperatures. [Carson & Cappellano, p87]

22   **c**   Alcohol may be disposed in the sewer system if it is a 24% or less dilution. [Carson & Cappellano, p93]

23   **b**   Total magnification is the magnification of the ocular multiplied by the magnification of the objective. [Carson & Cappellano, p54]

24   **a**   Class A fires involve wood and paper. [Carson & Cappellano, p91; Dapson, p217]

25   **d**   The iris diaphragm controls the amount of light on the slide. [Carson & Cappellano, p54]

26   **b**   Organic solvents cannot be disposed in the sewer system; therefore, they should be collected for distillation recovery or for a licensed waste hauler. [Carson & Cappellano, p93]

27   **c**   Use the percentage formula (%desired :100 = g or mL needed :volume desired) to calculate how to make the 1% acetic acid, and then how to make the 3% alcian blue in the acid. [Carson & Cappellano, p98]

28   **b**   350 mg is equivalent to 0.35 g. [Carson & Cappellano, p101]

29   **d**   Use the gravimetric factor formula (concentration of present dye ÷ concentration of new dye = gravimetric factor; then multiply the factor by the amount of dye required) to calculate the amount of new dye needed for the same concentration. [Carson & Cappellano, p99]

30   **c**   Phase contrast microscopes are used to examine living unstained tissues. [Carson & Cappellano, p56]

31   **d**   A buffer will resist change in pH. [Carson & Cappellano, p102]

32   **d**   The objective known as "high dry" is generally 45× magnification. [Carson & Cappellano, p54]

33   **b**   5 μm is equivalent to 0.005 mm in thickness. [Carson & Cappellano, p101]

34   **c**   The Material Safety Data Sheets are required by the Hazard Communication Act. [Dapson, p81]

35   **d**   Use the formula for diluting solutions that are less than 100% (beginning % × beginning volume = desired % × desired volume) for calculating the answer of 737 mL. [Carson & Cappellano, pp98-99]

36   **a**   Flammable liquids are required to be stored in flammable cabinets. [Dapson, p132]

37   **b**   Use the formula for diluting solutions that are less than 100% (beginning% × beginning volume = desired % × desired volume) for calculating the answer of 10 mL. [Carson & Cappellano, pp98-99]

38   **c**   Birefringent particles are doubly refractile. [Carson & Cappellano, p55]

39   **a**   Microwave energy causes rapid molecular movement which generates heat, and heat is a physical method of fixation. [Carson & Cappellano, pp2-3, 70]

40   **c**   Use the formula for diluting solutions that are less than 100% (beginning% × beginning volume = desired % × desired volume) for calculating the answer of 100 mL of water. [Carson & Cappellano, p98]

41 **b** Use the percentage formula (%desired :100 = g or mL needed :volume desired) for calculating the answer of 2.75 g. [Carson & Cappellano, p98]

42 **d** The NFPA blue area indicates health hazards, and the number 4 indicates an extreme health hazard. [Dapson, p125]

43 **a** Staining solutions used in the Warthin-Starry procedure must be pH 4; therefore, a buffer standard of pH 4 should be used to calibrate the pH meter. [Carson & Cappellano, p78]

44 **c** One cubic centimeter (cc) and one milliliter (mL) are equivalent and are often used interchangeably. [Carson & Cappellano, p101]

45 **c** The red quadrant of the NFPA diamond indicates flammability; the number 4 indicates extreme hazard, in this case easily ignited at room temperature. [Dapson, pp125, 132]

46 **d** 400 mm is equivalent to 40 cm. [Carson & Cappellano, p101]

47 **d** The definition of resolving power is the ability of a microscope to separate small details. [Carson & Cappellano, p54]

48 **b** Flammable liquid fires are classified as Class B fires. [Carson & Cappellano, p91; Dapson, p217]

49 **c** When a gallon of solvent is spilled, it may spread to an area of 20 square feet. [Carson & Cappellano, p90]

50 **c** Incineration must be used for disposing pathologic waste, according to the EPA. [Carson & Cappellano, p87]

51 **c** Micrometer pipettes are used primarily in immunohistochemistry procedures, and they need to have the calibration checked at least annually for accuracy. Pipettes as close to the volume needed should be chosen. [Carson & Cappellano, p79]

52 **b** A laboratory incubator is generally maintained at body temperature, 37°C. [Carson & Cappellano, p77]

53 **c** Robotic automated staining instruments allow exact times to be programmed for any given station. [Carson & Cappellano, p69]

54 **b** Use the formula for diluting solutions that are less than 100% (beginning% × beginning volume = desired % × desired volume) for calculating the answer of 3.45 mL. [Carson & Cappellano, p98]

55 **a** The formula for calculating percentage (w/v) is given in distractor a. [Carson & Cappellano, p98]

56 **d** Use the formula for diluting solutions that are less than 100% (beginning% × beginning volume = desired % × desired volume) for calculating the answer of 80 mL. [Carson & Cappellano, p98]

57 **c** The symbol shown indicates a biohazard. [Carson & Cappellano, p94]

58 **b** Solvents and contaminants boil off at various temperatures, and thus are separated. [Dapson, pp157-159]

59 **b** With longer exposure to microwave energy, the temperature increases. Thus to lower temperatures, decreasing the heating time is necessary. [Carson & Cappellano, pp2-3, 70]

60   **c**   Rotary microtomes are used for cutting paraffin blocks. [Carson & Cappellano, p58]

61   **d**   Use the formula for diluting solutions that are less than 100% (beginning% × beginning volume = desired % × desired volume) for calculating the answer of 50 mL. [Carson & Cappellano, p98]

62   **d**   Taking short breaks from repetitive motions will help prevent injuries. [Bancroft & Gamble, p669]

63   **c**   Polarizing microscopy utilizes both the polarizer film and an analyzer filter. [Carson & Cappellano, p55]

64   **c**   70 μm is equivalent to 0.07 mL. [Carson & Cappellano, p101]

65   **b**   Use the percentage formula (%desired :100 = g or mL needed :volume desired) for calculating the answer of 4%. [Carson & Cappellano, p98]

66   **b**   Use the percentage formula (%desired :100 = g or mL needed :volume desired) for calculating the answer of 200 mL. [Carson & Cappellano, p98]

67   **d**   The symbol shown indicates a flammable substance and protection from ignition sources is a must. [Carson & Cappellano, p94]

68   **b**   Acids may be disposed down the drain only if between pH 3 and pH 11. [Carson & Cappellano, p93]

69   **d**   Carbon dioxide fire extinguishers contain no water, and therefore are used on electrical fires. [Dapson, p217]

70   **b**   It is important to remove immersion oil promptly from the objectives, using lens paper only. [Bancroft & Gamble, p51; Carson & Cappellano, p54]

71   **a**   Because microwaves pass through glass and plastic containers, the liquid inside the container is heated but the container is not. [Carson & Cappellano, p70]

72   **d**   One μm (micron) is equivalent to 0.000001 meters. [Carson & Cappellano, p101]

73   **c**   Hydrochloric acid can cause extreme respiratory irritation, and should always be used under a ventilation hood. [Bancroft & Gamble, p28]

74   **b**   Chemical reactions take place more rapidly with an increase in temperature, as occurs with the microwave oven, thus taking less time than conventional processes. [Carson & Cappellano, p70]

75   **b**   Use the percentage formula (%desired :100 = g or mL needed :volume desired) for calculating the answer of 37.5 g. [Carson & Cappellano, p98]

76   **c**   Charged or plus slides, or ones with adhesive coating, will help sections adhere to the slides during subsequent procedures. [Carson & Cappellano, pp72-73]

77   **c**   Chronic repetitive trauma is a cause of the symptoms mentioned. [Bancroft & Gamble, p664]

78   **c**   LIS refers to the Laboratory Information System. [Carson & Cappellano, p330]

79   **b**   Polarizing microscopy is used to view the birefringence of amyloid after Congo red staining. [Carson & Cappellano, p55, 155]

80   **a**   The microscope condenser concentrates light on the tissue specimen. [Carson & Cappellano, p54]

81 **c** Paraffin wax is not considered a hazardous waste and can be put in the trash, unless it contains xylene. Paraffin waste from the embedding center would not contain xylene. [Dapson, p277]

82 **d** Automated cover slipping instrumentation will alleviate repetitive motion for that laboratory task, thus reducing the risk of injury. [Bancroft & Gamble, p670]

83 **c** Uranyl nitrate must be disposed by a licensed waste hauler. [Dapson, p277]

The following items (*) have been identified as more appropriate for entry level histotechnologists.

*84 **a** Use the formula for gravimetric factor (concentration of present dye ÷ concentration of new dye = gravimetric factor; then multiply the factor by the amount of dye required) for calculating the answer of 0.95 g. [Carson & Cappellano, p99]

*85 **a** Laboratory workers should never wear a "dirty" lab coat outside the lab. Management must re-train the employee in appropriate Bloodborne Pathogen Standard procedures. [Carson & Cappellano, pp86, 95]

*86 **b** Use the formula for Normal solution preparation (weight in grams = normality desired × volume desired in liters × formula weight ÷ positive valence) for calculating 5.55 g. [Carson & Cappellano, p100]

*87 **c** Use the formula for antibody dilution for calculating the answer of 20.0 mL. [Carson & Cappellano, p273]

*88 **a** Solutions containing mercury, chromium, or silver may not be disposed of in the sanitary sewer system. The other chemicals listed may be disposed down the drain. [Carson & Cappellano, p93; Dapson, p270]

*89 **d** The cognitive domain deals with the levels of understanding knowledge. [Harmening, pp154-155]

*90 **a** Because of the biohazardous waste in the cryostat, it must be disinfected before the equipment is serviced. [Carson & Cappellano, p67]

*91 **c** Use the formula for Molar solution preparation (weight in grams = molarity desired × volume × formula weight) to calculate the answer of 142.0 g. [Carson & Cappellano, p100]

*92 **c** Use the formula for the gravimetric factor (concentration of present dye ÷ concentration of new dye = gravimetric factor; then multiply the factor by the amount of dye required) for calculating the answer of 1.06 g. [Carson & Cappellano, p99]

*93 **b** When a teacher and student both know what learning outcomes are expected, the educational process is improved. [Harmening, pp158-159]

*94 **a** The polarizing microscope is used to view the Congo red stained slides for birefringence of amyloid deposits. [Brown, p134]

*95 **a** 100 µL is equivalent to 0.1 mL. [Carson & Cappellano, p101]

*96 **b** Verbs that are used in cognitive level one (recall of facts) include "define, describe, and identify." [Harmening, p156]

*97 **a** Plastic resins are known to produce contact dermatitis much more frequently than paraffin waxes. [Carson & Cappellano, p40]

*98 **a** This learning objective defines a psychomotor skill and to what degree the student would be expected to perform the skill. [Harmening, p157]

*99 **a** Use the formula for calculating Molar solutions (weight in grams = molarity desired × volume × formula weight) to determine the answer of 5 g. [Carson & Cappellano, p100]

*100 **c** Use the formula for antibody dilutions to calculate the answer of 20 μL. [Carson & Cappellano, p273]

*101 **c** NAACLS sets standards for, and accredits, histology laboratory training programs. [Harmening, p157]

*102 **d** Reduction of the use of chemicals is not a part of the planning process for handling chemical spills. [Dapson, p103]

*103 **c** Chloroform is categorized as a carcinogen, and requires safety precautions when it is used in the laboratory. [Carson & Cappellano, pp35, 90; Dapson, p240]

*104 **c** Tracer gas or smoke is the recommended method for initial testing of histology laboratory exhaust hoods. [Dapson, p112]

*105 **a** The EEO order is also called Affirmative Action. [Harmening, p95]

*106 **b** The ADEA protects people aged 40 and over from employment discriminations. [Harmening, pp107-108]

*107 **c** Each unit on the pH scale represents a 10-fold change in the concentration of hydronium ions. [Carson & Cappellano, p78]

*108 **c** During an employment interview, the candidate can only be asked job-related questions, never questions about his/her personal life. [Harmening, p120]

*109 **b** Performing tasks such as technical skills falls under the psychomotor objectives. [Harmening, p156]

*110 **c** Fire safety standards are prescribed by both OSHA and NFPA. [Dapson, p216]

*111 **b** Side-by-side comparisons are the best method of instrument validation. Controls and patient tissue, as appropriate, are handled identically through each step of the process, with the only variable being the "new" instrument. The final results are reviewed and approved by the laboratory medical director or designee. [Carson& Cappellano, p80]

*112 **d** Laboratory accreditation by the CAP is a voluntary peer review of laboratory processes and outcomes. [Harmening, p245]

*113 **c** Postanalytical refers to after the actual testing is done and the interpretation and reporting of results is being performed. [Harmening, p263]

*114 **a** When formaldehyde monitoring is done in the laboratory, results must be provided to employees within 15 days of the receipt of the results, according to the Formaldehyde Standard. [Carson & Cappellano, p90]

*115 **c** A competency performance evaluation is one in which the employee performs a task under the watch of a supervisor, to assure that the employee meets the established standards for the task. [Harmening, p121]

*116 **a** The spent amount is 33% more than the budgeted amount for overtime pay. [Harmening, p215]

*117 **c** The formula for calculating a Normal solution is given. [Carson & Cappellano, p100]

*118 **b** The formula for calculating gram equivalent weight of a chemical is given. [Carson & Cappellano, p100]

*119 **d** Thioflavin T is a fluorescent stain, and slides stained with it must be examined by a fluorescence microscope. [Carson & Cappellano, p157]

*120 **a** Use the formula for antibody dilution for calculating the answer of a 1:5 dilution. [Carson & Cappellano, p273]

*121 **c** The position description is the document that describes the duties of a particular job position in the laboratory. [Harmening, pp97-100]

*122 **d** All new instrumentation must be validated before put into use for patient samples. [Carson & Cappellano, p80]

*123 **c** The red quadrant of the NFPA label indicates flammability, and a number 3 indicates that the liquid will easily ignite. [Dapson, p125]

*124 **c** The substage condenser functions primarily to concentrate light on the tissue section. [Carson & Cappellano, p54]

*125 **c** 40 hours per week for 50 weeks equals 2,080 total hours worked by a full time employee (FTE). [Harmening, p354]

*126 **b** To increase the light on the specimen when changing objectives, open the iris diaphragm. [Bancroft & Gamble, p37; Carson & Cappellano, p54]

*127 **a** The formula for calculating Molar solutions is given. [Carson & Cappellano, p100]

*128 **c** Use the formula for diluting solutions that are <100% (beginning% × beginning volume = desired % × desired volume) for calculating the answer of 3,529.40 mL. [Carson & Cappellano, p98]

*129 **a** Objectives should be measurable by testing so that it can be determined if the student has achieved the objective of the lesson. [Harmening, p158]

*130 **b** Mercury is not used in most histology laboratories because of the hazards it presents. [Dapson, p257]

*131 **b** The Formaldehyde Standard sets the TWA to be no more than 0.75 ppm, so the ventilation system must be able to meet that standard. [Carson & Cappellano, p89; Dapson, p22]

*132 **a** The technician is showing signs of contact dermatitis commonly seen with latex sensitivity. [Dapson, pp78, 129]

*133 **c** If monitoring reveals a level above 0.5 ppm, re-monitoring is required within 6 months. [Carson & Cappellano, p89]

*134 **a** Dependability in attendance is an affective behavior. [Harmening, p157]

*135 **a** Collagen is autofluorescent, and therefore would be visualized when viewing a FITC stained section. [Carson & Cappellano, p56]

*136 **b** The numerical aperture of a microscope objective indicates its resolving power. [Bancroft & Gamble, p38]

*137 **b** A quality assurance program focuses on laboratory processes in order to assure a quality final product. [Bancroft & Gamble, p4]

*138 **b** Cognitive, or thought processes, are the focus of Bloom's Taxonomy. Levels from beginner to expert are assigned. [Harmening, p154]

*139 **b** In an employment interview, only inquiries regarding the applicant's ability to meet the requirements of the position are allowed. [Harmening, p120]

*140 **c** The job (or position) description defines the role of an employee in a given position in the laboratory. [Harmening, pp99-100]

*141 **b** The straight-line depreciation formula is used to calculate the depreciation of an instrument. [Harmening, p202]

*142 **c** Dividing the total labor hours by 2,080 (amount of hours per FTE), results in 6.1 FTE. [Harmening, p354]

*143 **b** Certification indicates that a person has met the minimal standard for entry level knowledge and skills for a profession, usually by a testing method. The ASCP Board of Certification sets the certification requirements, and grants certification (HT, HTL) to persons who qualify for and successfully pass the certification examination. [Harmening]

*144 **b** The objective is in the Cognitive domain, as it expects the student to be able to recall facts (knowledge). [Harmening, p158]

*145 **c** HIPAA (Health Insurance Portability & Accountability Act) is concerned with patient privacy. [Carson &Cappellano, p333]

*146 **b** Although an OSHA standard was passed regarding ergonomics in the workplace in 2001, it was repealed later that same year. There is currently no regulation regarding ergonomics. [Carson & Cappellano, p88]

*147 **c** Any new antibody received into the laboratory must be validated before use on patient samples for diagnosis. [Carson & Cappellano, pp272-273]

*148 **c** Psychomotor objectives deal with learning to perform a technical skill or task such as microtomy. [Harmening, p157]

*149 **d** The NSH/CAP HistoQIP reviews slides from laboratories in a voluntary, peer reviewed educational program for improvement of quality across laboratories. [Bancroft & Gamble, p5]

*150 **a** The periodic acid used as the oxidizer in the periodic acid-methenamine silver procedure seen in the image can be disposed into the sanitary sewer system. [Dapson, p264]

*151 **d** Paperless procedure manuals are not a part of barcoding. They are a separate electronic file. [Carson & Cappellano, p333-335]

*152 **a** Staining protocols are found in either an electronic or printed copy of the laboratory procedure manual, and are not concerned with bar codes. [Carson & Cappellano, pp333-335]

*153 **c** Pictograms are required on chemical labels (both commercial and in-house preparations) under the revised Hazard Communication Standard (revised in 2012). [Carson & Cappellano, p93]

*154 **b** Signal words, along with pictograms, and a chemical hazard statement are required under the revised Hazard Communication Standard (Hazard Communication 2012). [Carson& Cappellano, p93]

Reading & References

General Histotechnology

Bancroft JD, Gamble M [2008] *Theory & Practice of Histological Techniques, 6th ed*. New York, NY: Churchill Livingstone. ISBN:978-0443102790.

Brown RW, ed [2009] *Histologic Preparations: Common Problems & Their Solutions*. Northfield, IL: College of American Pathologists. ISBN:978-0930304959.

Carson F, Cappellano C [2015] *Histotechnology: A Self-Instructional Text, 4th ed*. Chicago, IL: ASCP Press. ISBN:978-0891896319.

Dapson JC, Dapson RW [1995] *Hazardous Materials in the Histopathology Laboratory, 4th ed*. Battle Creek, MI: Anatech. ISBN:978-0964519701.

Kiernan J [2010] *Histological and Histochemical Methods: Theory & Practice, 4th ed*. Oxfordshire, England: Scion Publishing. ISBN:978-1904842422.

Young B, Lowe JS, et al [2006] *Wheater's Functional Histology: A Text & Colour Atlas, 5th ed*. New York, NY: Churchill Livingstone. ISBN:978-0443068508.

Management & Education

Harmening DM [2007] *Laboratory Management: Principles & Processes, 2nd ed*. St Petersburg, FL: DH Publishing & Consulting. ISBN:978-0803615991.

ISBN 978-089189-6494   ©ASCP 2016

rosebud